I0039162

REGISTER TODAY

FOR ADDITIONAL BONUSES!

Visit

www.IAmBishop.com/ThinkFactor

When you register on-line you receive access to one month of on-line coaching from me personally and access to my special fitness and lifestyle tools, including three complete individualized programs that will guide your progress. You can register anytime by visiting *www.IAmBishop.com/ThinkFactor.*

THE
THINK
FACTOR

You Are Fitter Than You Think

BRENT BISHOP

BOUND
PUBLISHING

Copyright © 2011 By Brent Bishop
This book may not be reproduced in whole or in part, by any means, without written consent of the publisher.

Bound Publishing

United States
6501 E. Greenway Pkwy
#103-480
Scottsdale, AZ
85254

Canada
Suite 114
720 28th St. NE
Calgary, AB T2A 6R3

Toll Free Phone and Fax: 1-888-237-1627
Email: info@boundpublishing.com
Web: www.boundpublishing.com

ISBN: 978-0-9867762-0-5

Cover & Text: Anamarie Seidel; Finely Finished LLC
Edit: Lynda Masterson; Valyn Enterprises LLC
Interior Photography: LA Wade
Back Cover Photography: Rob De Franco, www.RobDeFranco.com

COMPANIES, ORGANIZATIONS, INSTITUTIONS, AND INDUSTRY PUBLICATIONS. Quantity discounts are available on bulk purchases of this book for reselling, educational purposes, subscription incentives, gifts, sponsorship, or fundraising. Special books or book excerpts can also be created to fit specific needs such as private labeling with your logo on the cover and a message from a VIP printed inside. For more information, please contact our Special Sales Department at Bound Publishing.

TABLE OF
CONTENTS

Dedication

I have been blessed with the company of inspirational people, continued support, amazing opportunities and perspectives that have truly helped shape and form who I am today. If it were not for those individuals, I am confident my success level would not be nearly as great as it is today. I would like to mention a few individuals who profoundly influenced my life and work.

First and foremost, I dedicate this book to Lauriann Wade. Without her unwavering support, inspiration, constant accountability and contribution in my personal and professional life, this book and concept would have not been possible. She encapsulates a true example of just how powerful the relationship between mindset and fitness can be in personal reinvention and optimal performance.

To my parents: two of the most kind, generous and selfless people I know. They not only provided a safe and loving environment for me growing up, but also continue to be the number-one supporters of anything I choose to do in life. They have given me the confidence, freedom and curiosity to not only *let* life happen, but to also *make* life happen.

To my close friends: I have many acquaintances but few truly close friends. These friends have always supported my decisions, shown interest in me and, although we now live far apart, have always made time to stay connected.

To my team at Think Fitness: my career would not be where it is today without the professional, passionate and enthusiastic team at Think Fitness. Without them my passion for inspiring others through fitness would be unfulfilled. I have been truly blessed with an amazing management, marketing, administrative and training team who share my core values and the passion for inspiring communities.

To my clients: those whom I have trained and influenced but more importantly, those who have also influenced me. There isn't one client with whom I have worked over the years of personal training who has not influenced me in some way. Every interaction, every story and every personality has provided me with great insight into how human beings operate; what holds them back, what inspires them and how to help them tap into their true potential. They have also been a mirror into my own obstacles, weaknesses and strengths, which has allowed me to continue my own quest towards my life purpose and passion.

My deep gratitude goes out to you all!

About The Author

Brent Bishop is an entrepreneur, actor, author and highly sought after personal trainer and lifestyle coach. This renowned fitness expert is the owner of Think Fitness Studios™, a performance-inspired, boutique personal training center in Toronto. He is also the regular Fitness Expert on CTV's The Marilyn Denis Show and Functional Fitness Host of the series Body Fuel.

Bishop holds a B.Sc. in Kinesiology with a minor in Psychology from Simon Fraser University, British Columbia. He has over 16 years of experience inspiring people of all levels to demand more of themselves through fitness. Bishop has notable fitness career highlights working with Olympians, high level athletes and various film and television personalities.

Whether it's hiking the Andes in Peru, leading a group on a snowshoeing expedition or planning his next eco-adventure race, Bishop dedicates his time and energy to inspire himself and others to realize their true potential by unleashing their inner athlete.

THE THINK FACTOR

PREFACE

It was 5:45 am on a cold Tuesday morning. I was standing at Bev's front door. As a personal trainer who is perhaps excessively passionate about the wellbeing of his clients, I was worried. Bev (not her real name) was slipping. She was giving up on the health and fitness goals she had set for herself just a couple of months earlier.

I was about to call on her, uninvited, to try to pull her back on the wagon. As a child and younger adult Bev had been an active recreational athlete. However children, job responsibilities, shifting priorities and the general busyness of life had had a profound effect on how she viewed herself as the years passed.

Now middle-aged, she had gained 50 pounds and her self-image had begun a downward spiral of self-pity and self-destruction. In terms of her health, physical fitness and self-image, Bev was entering what I—with more than 15 years experience as a kinesiologist and coach—had come to recognize was a cycle of self-destruction. She had come to the realization that she was not as fit as she should be, but had lost the conviction that she could do anything about it. What's more, she had lost her enthusiasm for the effort to get back in physical and emotional shape. She needed an external force to get her back on track.

A couple of months before, Bev had come to me exhibiting the unfortunate symptoms of a mid-life period of inactivity—what I have come to call the "mid-life fitness crisis". I was not her first coach. A few years earlier she had summoned up the courage to hire another personal trainer to help her lose weight and increase her activity level.

She candidly shared her experience with me. She would wake up early and go to the gym where she felt like an outsider—a washed-up, has-been ex-sports enthusiast who was now a self conscious "fat person", lacking the coordination, confidence and fitness to become healthy and normal again.

Her experience with her previous personal trainer had taught her about accountability, and she was smart enough to instinctively realize that her previously healthy life was slipping. She had lasted about two months with the other trainer and then fallen off the fitness wagon just as she was beginning to change her bad habits. She said her training routine had become physically and mentally predictable and she no longer felt challenged. Human nature is like that.

Bev resumed her former lifestyle, characterized by inactivity and self-defeat. She essentially gave up; thinking "what's the point, why bother"? Soon she was again convinced that she was just another "fat person". Eventually, however, she realized that she was in a rut, and although she was never going to be a competitive athlete, her real problem was attitude. She simply had lost the spark that used to get her fired up about being active.

I recalled Bev telling me about this during our initial consultation. For a couple of weeks I had been watching her increasingly lose interest and begin to regress. I knew this was the crisis point. Either I give up on her completely or give her her a big jolt of reality. I decided to give her the jolt.

Bev's condition is fairly common among middle-aged busy adults. Its symptoms are lack of activity, increased weight gain and feelings of unworthiness and self-pity. I couldn't be easy on her if I wanted her to overcome that. So although I knew I was taking a big risk by pushing her so hard, I wasn't about to let go. If I let her slip back now, without even trying to help, I would never forgive myself.

So here I was at 5:45 am in front of her house, ignoring the fact that she had e-mailed me an excuse explaining why she couldn't make it to her session.

My plan was to respectfully, but sternly, show her that I cared about her, and to make her see just how close she was to real change without realizing it. All she saw was the easy way out—the way she was accustomed to, the journey she felt most comfortable with. Once again she had reached the threshold of challenge and her next step would determine the outcome. My job was to show her what was possible if she worked outside her comfort zone once again.

In doing so, I believed she would see that each uncomfortable challenge is merely another step towards the person she really wanted to be, and thus regain that athletic drive she had experienced years before. I could see it so strongly that I was determined not to give up on her, and not to let her give up on herself.

I'll never forget the expression on her face when she opened the door that morning. She was used to coming to see me at the gym and being in control. This was about to change. The look on her face was somewhere between furious and embarrassed. Having backed out of the session, she was moping around the house before getting ready to go to work.

"Get dressed in your workout gear, our workout is outside today," I said.

With no excuses left, she poured me a glass of water and went off to change into her workout clothes. When we set off, there was nothing but awkward silence.. Eventually, as we continued to jog down the street, she started to become more cordial. During our jog to a nearby park she voiced what had been going on in her head. That she had hit the wall—the mid-life fitness crisis.

From that day forward, until Bev took a job out of the country, we had four years of unbelievable progress. Bev went through continual personal challenge and accountability and proved that by participating in an interest-driven program, she would continue to succeed. Today she is really an athlete. She's in better shape than she has been since she was a teenager. Her confidence is unmatched and her success in life very admirable. It was always in her—present but hidden—encapsulated by feelings of uselessness, age and mediocrity.

Professional athlete, successful entrepreneur or full time mom, everyone needs a change at some point in his or her life. I was glad to initiate the change that Bev seemed to need during this time.

Her story is one of many that have inspired me, as a professional in the health, lifestyle and fitness industry, to realize that all of us have a trigger—something within us that, when unleashed, can have a powerful impact on our lives. Sometimes all it takes is that one crucial element that gets us out of a rut and propels us forward—the "Think Factor".

Physical exercise combined with purposeful challenge and healthy thinking can be an amazing recipe that reveals that which truly maximizes the potential within us.

So read on. Take your time. Complete the suggested exercises as you read through the chapters. Determine how this concept—and the exercises that go with it—can be used to consistently produce results and maximize *your* potential. Whether you are looking to jumpstart your fitness routine, or feel you are at a standstill with regard to your health and fitness, you need to take your game to the next level.

The Think Factor will help make it happen for you.

Fit Tip

AND HERE'S AN ADDED BONUS!

Visit
www.IAmBishop.com/ThinkFactor

When you register on-line you receive access to one month of on-line coaching from me personally and access to my special fitness and lifestyle tools, including three complete individualized programs that will guide your progress. You can register anytime by visiting *www.IAmBishop.com/ThinkFactor*

Chapter One

ABANDONING MEDIOCRITY[1]

'Mediocrity is the refuge
of the unimaginative and uninspired.'
~ ANONYMOUS

MEDIOCRITY (NOUN)
1. Ordinariness as a consequence of being average and not outstanding
2. A person of second-rate ability or value

Media...Mediocrity...coincidence? I think not. In this age of media-driven existence, mediocrity often spells disaster in many people's lives. With companies telling us how to dress, what to eat, what cars to drive and even where to live, we are surrounded by a suffocating blanket of mediocrity that leaves us unwilling to think for ourselves and be productive, assertive citizens. Too many people today just plug along in life thinking and doing only what so-called "experts" in the media tell us is appropriate.

> *The general tendency of things throughout the world is to render mediocrity the ascendant power among mankind.*
> ~ JOHN STUART MILL

The "lemming like" way of living that too many people have succumbed to, is almost exclusively driven by technology— what I call the bane of human activity. Technology is wonderful as a tool but shouldn't eliminate activity and real human connection. With the age of television, the personal computer, the Internet, and social media such as Facebook and Twitter, millions of formerly active, busy people now lapse into lethargy as they sit for hours in front of their monitors. So technology is not only telling us how to live, but too often technology is also doing that living for us. Our fast paced technological society is rendering us mediocre.

Whenever a large sample of chaotic elements are taken in hand and marshalled in the order of their magnitude, an unsuspected and most beautiful form of regularity proves to have been latent all along.

Francis Galton refers to this as the "Supreme Law of Unreason". In plain English, it means when you take a group of average active people, give them technology and feed them all the "answers" to life's questions, they descend into mediocrity. They stop challenging themselves and their sense of curiosity, spontaneity, and adventure regresses.

Take Citizen Joe for example. He wakes up every morning to the sound of the commercials (interrupted occasionally by musical selections) on his radio alarm clock. Then he shuffles off to the bathroom to shower, shave and brush his teeth using products recommended on television by nine out of ten specialists. After rummaging through his wardrobe for the brand name clothes that he bought because that's what everyone is wearing nowadays, he goes downstairs to breakfast on his "favorite" brand of cereal—the one he saw advertised last week on a television commercial which informed him that it contains every nutritional thing he needs to start his day.

After breakfast, it's off to his cubicle at Consolidated Widget, where he sits in front of his computer from 9:00 to 5:00 before coming home to catch up on the work he didn't have time to complete at the office. He does this Monday thru Friday, has no energy left on the weekends and, is only vaguely aware of the mundane and mediocre loop that he has drifted into.

The sad thing is that it wouldn't take much to change Joe's way of life back from Flab to Fab—all he needs to do is discover one thing in his life that he is passionate about, and he would accomplish a lot more without much additional effort. Matching his passion with an activity that gets him moving would have the power to catapult his daily routine in a new and positive direction.

The problem is that Joe, like lots of people, is afraid to live outside the box. He's accustomed to spending his life in a mediocre comfort zone of minimum effort. If you asked him if he had any other goal in life he probably wouldn't have a clear and direct answer, because he doesn't think he could achieve it even if he did.

I say all Joe really needs is a change of mindset. Right now he just jumps in and follows the crowd. How much more rewarding do you think his life would be if he gave some thought to what he really wanted, and deliberately set out to make that happen, regardless of what others are doing. Creating change in our lives is ninety percent mental. It's not that difficult. However, initiating change requires inspiration. The key to becoming inspired is to take charge of your own life.

Accountability is the vital trait that enables us to move beyond mediocrity and start achieving extraordinary results. The trouble is that many people get stuck in seemingly inescapable ruts and try to find relief, even if it is only temporary. Instead the blame others for their unhappiness. They refuse to take responsibility for their inadequacies, instead blaming their lack of education, their upbringing, their employer, the economy, the government—the list goes on and on. However it doesn't really matter who or what they blame, because placing the responsibility outside of themselves means that they don't have to assume personal control over their lives. The single most outstanding characteristic of successful people is that they accept responsibility for themselves and refuse to blame others for their condition in life.

Taking responsibility begins by accepting the fact that—at the end of the day—you are the only one who is really accountable for who you are. However, many fail to see that achieving accountability is a process. You need to do it every day.

Every day all of us are faced with decisions that need to be made, and obligations that must be agreed upon or kept. These include everything from getting up in the morning and choosing to go into work, to things like whether to stay in a particular marriage or job, or choose what career to pursue.

It becomes very easy and appealing to continue putting off until tomorrow those things that we find tedious, hard or uncomfortable today. Before we know it, weeks, months, even years have gone by and our dreams remain unfulfilled. As the disappointments and frustrations mount, it becomes a vicious cycle. It becomes more difficult to accept responsibility for a life that has deteriorated into mediocrity.

The good news is that it is never too late to make a positive change. Every day offers a new chance to start over, to take charge of your life, to become accountable for who you are. You don't have to change your entire way of living. All you need to do is change one thing, and you'll see how your thoughts on life will change and, in turn, change the way you live the rest of your life.

It's really not all that difficult to rise above mediocrity, but it does require persistence. Here are five simple steps that will help you:

1. HAVE A DREAM

Having a dream gives you something to strive for. If you're one of those people who go through life thinking that dreaming is a silly waste of time and that dreams are too hard to accomplish in real life, you're never going to get anywhere. That kind of thinking is what keeps so many people in a state of mediocrity. Only a comparative few are willing to follow their dreams to achieve more than the status quo.

I say dream—dream big—and go after those dreams with everything you are.

2. DON'T BE ONE OF THE CROWD

If you want to get beyond the mediocre, and start getting excellent results, you have to break free of the crowd and do things differently than everyone else is doing. For example, instead of going to your gym every morning and running on the treadmill, go out for a jog around your neighborhood. You'll get far more enjoyment by being outdoors, watching the scenery go by, enjoying the fresh air and listening to the comments of encouraging onlookers. Changing something this simple is all it takes to get you another step farther from mediocrity. Making a point of changing your daily, weekly routine on a regular basis can keep things interesting and have profound effects on your lifestyle.

3. BREAK FREE OF YOUR SAFETY ZONE

Too many people nowadays are afraid to step outside their comfort zones. However by staying within these artificial boundaries they are losing out on great opportunities to skyrocket to that next level of success. So what if the tasks before you are uncomfortable. They're supposed to be hard. The "hard" is what makes them beneficial. If you want to learn to swim you have to be willing to get your feet wet!

4. CHALLENGE YOURSELF

By avoiding hard tasks, you condemn yourself to living in a rut. When you stay within your comfort zones you start to slack off.

Things that are worth doing are the very things that are hard to do at first, but they will also provide you with the greatest rewards. So challenge yourself to do something new, and difficult, and you'll step out of the box that is mediocrity.

5. GO AFTER WHAT YOU REALLY WANT

Never settle for anything less than what you really want. If you do, you'll never end up with the big prize. Why? Because the big prizes never go to those who give up too soon. So work hard, persevere, and don't settle for less. You will get what you want.

Fit Tip

Tomorrow, choose one thing to do differently. Make sure it is positive and leads you in the direction of who you want to become. It could be something as simple as having a balanced breakfast in the morning, or making a point of drinking eight glasses of water each day, or waking up a half-hour earlier than you did today in order to get some exercise.

Whether you are a novice just beginning to make exercise and fitness part of your life, or a recreational athlete trying to get that additional edge for your sport, there is always something that you can tweak or implement. This will not only change the stimulus you get from it, but also change the way you think about your health, goals and fitness—your mindset.

REMEMBER

When you register on-line you receive access to one month of on-line coaching from me personally and access to my special fitness and lifestyle tools, including three complete individualized programs that will guide your progress. You can register anytime by visiting *www. IAmBishop.com/ThinkFactor*

Chapter Two

RAISING THE BAR

Having gotten yourself out of the rut of mediocrity, it's time to raise the bar to the next level by setting more challenging goals and starting the hard-but-satisfying work of achieving them. Remember, nobody said moving beyond mediocrity is going to be easy, but the rewards will surely justify the effort.

In order to set your new goals, you must first examine your current life in detail and consider what behaviors you will need to modify. This will allow you to let go of the way you are currently living and start living the healthy life that you've envisioned for yourself.

Here's a tip—this is too big a process to attempt in a single step. You need to break it down into a series of short-term changes—each with its own goal—that will enable you to move toward your new life one step at a time. Breaking down the process into short-term goals not only gives you a way to check your progress but also keeps you motivated. Believe it or not, this actually makes it physically and emotionally easier to achieve your goal of a healthier, happier and more fulfilling life. We will expand further on the process of effective goal setting in the chapters to come.

EXAMINING YOUR PRESENT LIFESTYLE

We human beings are extremely adept at the process of learning. When you come to think about it, that's one of the main advantages we have over other members of the animal kingdom. Elephants are stronger, horses are faster, dogs have a keener sense of smell and hearing, butterflys are more beautiful, ants are more prolific, and even the simplest of bacteria are more durable. Our unique ability, to make logical decisions, to know right from wrong, to decide what we should do to be healthy, and to reason out how to make things happen is the essence of our species.

However, knowing alone is not enough. Being educated on what to eat, what are healthy decisions versus unhealthy decisions, or what exercises to do to optimize your workout time, simply become academic if we don't do anything about it.

For example, we all know that overeating is unhealthy, but millions of people still fall victim to obesity. If we're so smart, why does that happen? Of course, there can be several reasons—not everyone has access to the right kinds of foods can be one; lack of knowledge regarding what foods are or are not good for us may be another. But in our society, perhaps the most common reasons are (i) we have too many choices—not all of which are good for us, (ii) eating has become a stress-reduction strategy in our increasingly stressed-out society, and (iii) we are constantly bombarded by media messages urging us to eat this, that, or the other thing. In moderation, they may be good for us but taken in combination—or in excess—can be hazardous to our health.

We may intellectually know the right things to do, but the media, stress and experiences of life are constantly sending us messages that try to persuade us differently. These messages— repeated day after day, month after month, year after year— eventually play a major role in forming the reflexive habits we manifest in our lives.

Habits are individually learned activities, as opposed to instincts, which are characteristics of an entire species. You cannot do things habitually unless you have learned to do them and you cannot learn a habit without repetition. The more the repetition, the deeper the habit becomes ingrained. The more that societal and other external forces reinforce these learned habits, the harder they are to break. People learn to become overweight or unhealthy—it doesn't just happen.

Human beings do what we learn. Changing life patterns that hold us back requires that we replace these patterns with newly learned behaviors that move us forward. This begins by implementing a series of small positive changes that move us in the direction we want to go.

The way to do this is a technique known as reflexive learning. Reflexive learning is identifying something you already know. For example: you know that starting every day with a balanced breakfast is a healthy eating habit. Now create a plan that allows you to repeat the action you want to become a habit. Continue to repeat that action without fail for as long as it takes for it to become an unconscious habit. This will probably require less time than you expect. When the laws requiring the use of seat belts in cars came into effect, there were millions of people who truly believed they would never remember to buckle up. However, subsequent studies confirmed that the average person acquired the habit in about three weeks.

So start by identifying what you already know about healthy living.

CREATING AND IMPLEMENTING AN ACTION PLAN

An action plan is much more than just a schedule of daily tasks. It is also a tool to keep us focused and motivated. A plan that keeps reminding us of who we are and why we are here. This prevents us from forgetting our purpose and losing interest in achieving our goals. An action plan must be interesting, inspiring, highly purposeful and of course, action oriented. This is where creativity comes into play.

It is not enough, for example, to determine that you want to lose weight. You have to specify exactly how much weight you want to lose, within what time frame you want to lose it, what milestones you will reach during that time frame and, most importantly, why you want to lose it and what you will feel like afterwards. The more descriptive your overall vision is, the more drive you will have to achieve your goal. How to develop an effective action plan for your goals will be addressed later in this book.

THE MENTAL MUSCLE

The mind is a mental muscle. Like the body's physical muscles, the mind requires consistent exercise for optimal performance. Education, interactive conversation, brainstorming, conscious thinking—all of these are essential in any training modality. Learning to take control of the way your mind works—your mindset—is how you truly harness the power to achieve. This is an important concept to grasp.

At Think Fitness™ Studios, my personalized fitness training facility in Toronto, our team of professionals utilize this concept to maximize our clients' ability to achieve life-changing results. Think Fitness™ is an important concept that combines mental fitness with physical fitness. Our goal is to teach and inspire all our clients—through a holistic fitness experience—to take control of their mindsets. This will purposefully expand their comfort zones in order to achieve optimal performance.

One hour can make all the difference between **good performance** and **great performance.** The writer who spends an extra 60 minutes a day honing his craft will see improvements spill out of his pen. A college student who devotes 60 additional minutes to study each day will cement her name on the honor roll. It is amazing what you can accomplish just by asking a bit more of yourself.

It isn't difficult to work an extra hour of effort into your day. If you can't put in all the time at once, you can split it into 30-minute or even 15-minute segments. You will also be amazed at how effectively this can eliminate many time-wasting activities that you perform each day. This will help you replace them with healthier activities that will get you closer to your fitness goal.

When we ask more of ourselves, we tend to rise to the occasion and grow. Conversely, if we get too comfortable we stagnate.

The essence of habit formation is simply to devote a certain amount of time each day to the formation of any habit you wish to establish, and do it faithfully for a specified number of consecutive days. At the end of this habit formation period, it should actually be harder **not** to engage in the new behaviour than it would be to continue it. This applies to any type of habit, from a physical practice to changing your self-image in the theatre of your mind.

The Think Fitness Program uses a Quarterly Habit Forming System, wherein 90 days is seen as the amount of time required to see significant results and create some momentum for positive changes. This will also help to establish habituation if the behaviour. For this reason, it is helpful to perform your exercises at the same time every day.

Other senses can also be utilized to establish a habit. If you want to establish the habit of meditating you can reinforce it by wearing the same clothing, burning the same incense, being in the same location and assuming the same posture at the same time every day for 21 consecutive days. This is another common habit-forming time frame. If you miss a day, just keep going until you've been doing the new behaviour for 21 days.

The more senses you involve in creating the new habit, the more deeply it will become ingrained in your self-image. So try to use all the faculties of your imagination. Include sights, sounds, smells, emotions and taste to strengthen the picture that you want to associate with your new self-image. In other words, make it as real as possible.

Research has indicated that different lengths of time are required for the formation of different habits. In the end, however, it all boils down to learning how to form habits—healthy habits—and make practical decisions that you can actually implement.

Now, as you are developing a better understanding of how to shift your focus toward developing new positive behaviors into habits, it is time to take action. But, before you do, think about it. Most people go through life in a comfort zone of bare minimum. Now that you have a general understanding of an action plan, you can start to *Think Fitness.*

Getting and staying fit is 10 percent physical and 90 percent mental! Inspiration is not simply the process of getting excited and rushing off, expecting to achieve your goals in any way possible. It's a lot more complicated than that. However complexity is never a hindrance if you understand it.

Fit Tip

Create an Inspiration Identity Worksheet to brainstorm what's going to motivate you to change.

1. On a piece of paper or on your computer, create three columns

2. Title the left column: **A - What I Am**

3. Title the middle column: **B - What I Want To Be**

4. Title the right column: **Getting From A to B**

5. Over the next week, write down all the things you are in the left column and what you want to be in the middle column.

6. In the right column, list those aspects of your current life that inspire you and what aspects work against that inspiration. Those aspects of your life might be physical or mental.

7. Start doing more of those things that do motivate you and fewer of the things that work against that motivation.

REMEMBER TO VISIT

www.IAmBishop.com/ThinkFactor

You'll receive access to useful worksheets, training guides, additional fitness programs and exclusive access to Brent Bishop for one month of free on-line coaching!

Chapter Three

YOUR LIFE STRATEGY

There is a distinct difference between *fitness* as it relates to lifestyle and the general idea of *exercise*, which is traditionally seen as something we have to do to stay healthy.

"My doctor told me I have to exercise," "I need to exercise to lose weight," "I want to look good for my wedding so I know I need to exercise."

These are all very common thoughts when it comes to exercise. They reflect a mindset that views exercise as something we should do or have to do.

My concept of fitness is quite different. To me, fitness relates to wellness, longevity, getting the most out of your life, functionality, and new experiences that are truly life changing.

Fitness is power, confidence, vitality, performance and excitement—all the things we all want out of life. Yet many people still have a mental disconnect when it comes to what physical fitness can do for them.

My childhood years were spent in Prince George, British Columbia where being active, enjoying life outdoors, hiking and biking were the norm. It wasn't until I became an adult that I realized just how many people take their physical bodies for granted when it comes to day-to-day living.

More importantly, as I grew up I also realized how taking your physical body for granted can detract from your mental state, reduce your confidence, energy, and ability to handle stress, and affect the overall balance of your life. What was missing from many people's lives was that sense of play; the inner need to move and be continually active.

Traditionally, becoming fit means working—the entire concept revolves around physical exercise. However in my personal experience, working for over 16 years with a wide variety of people of all ages, I have come to realize that good physical health can provide a powerful influence on most of the key aspects our lives. Conversely, poor physical health can have an equally adverse effect.

Growing up in Western Canada, living and working in Vancouver, British Columbia and the west coast of California, I came to the realization at a young age that it was extremely important to my personal well being to get outside and run, bike and hike the trails of the Rocky Mountains on a regular basis—it kept me feeling alive, focused and continually inspired.

On the relatively few occasions when I took a break from this lifestyle, I found something wasn't right. I would become stressed-out and irritated more easily, and my focus and mental perception of myself as well as those around me were negatively impacted.

As I studied and worked to become a fitness professional, these personal experiences led me to look at others who had not grown up with the outdoor experience, or had never experienced the mental contrast between active and inactive lifestyles.

I have come to a fundamental conclusion about life in a largely urban society. The larger and more industrialized a city is, the more the people living and working there get busier and busier. This results in more stressors for them and increased demands on their time, in order to keep up the pace of that lifestyle. This is hardly surprising, but its implications were very significant to me as a young fitness professional.

I began to understand that it is even more important to have a physical fitness routine when one lives in a big city than it is if one lives in a rural area. Because the unhealthy stresses of life in the city can be greater than those in the country, a fitness routine becomes a means of balancing your life.

Early in my training and coaching career, I found myself trying to use what I call "power of contrast." This helps people realize what they could achieve if they would demand more of themselves and explore the unfamiliar. When people are provided with a distinct change in stimulus—one that provides a real contrast to their current lifestyle—powerful changes can occur.

By continuing to place themselves in new and, perhaps uncomfortable situations, people begin to redefine what is "comfortable" for them. It may only be a slight change—a new view of their personal capabilities perhaps, or a tiny step in strengthening their mind. That is what is most important to them, because it can broaden their perspective and cause them to grow, if only a little bit. That's what is most important—to create this contrast regularly in our lives keeps us growing. Constant growth is essential to good health.

My fiancé Lauriann Wade is an incredibly perceptive and inquisitive life coach. There are powerful similarities and differences in our approaches. When I met Lauriann she had never been the "workout" type. She never really liked going to a gym and definitely was not a runner. But she has an unsurpassed ability to see people for who they are and to tap into the "mental" aspects of what is holding them back.

Early in our relationship it was evident my concept of physical fitness and her concept of mental fitness resulted in personal growth for both of us. Lauriann's self-reflection process was a source of strength for me. Lauriann was strengthened by the impact that purposeful exercise had on her life. The combination of our philosophies led us both to a whole new model of living.

THE PERFORMANCE CONTINUUM PARADIGM©

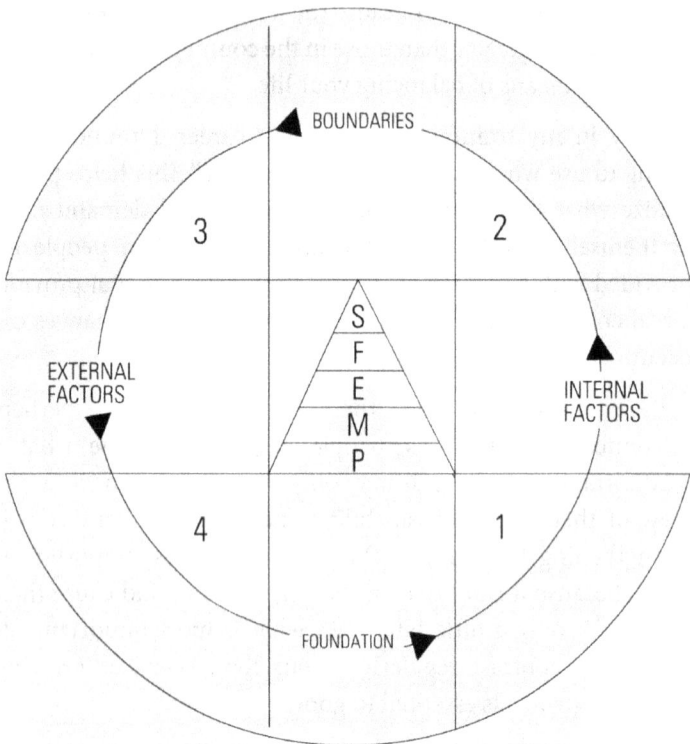

The Performance Continuum Paradigm© is a practical guide to optimal performance. This model comes from the concepts of both mental and physical fitness. People often attempt to separate these two concepts, but I've come to realize that this is virtually impossible. As co-creators of this paradigm, Lauriann and I have used it both personally and professionally, witnessing firsthand its powerful results.

Your mental state determines how you present yourself in the world. The old saying, "what you fill your mind with, you will be" is both timeless and true. However, your mental state (or mindset) is greatly influenced by your physical health. When you align the two, the results can be well beyond your initial expectations. The key is to hold yourself accountable for following the plan you make.

Professionally, my goal is to teach and inspire people around the world to enhance their lives through health and fitness. This goal has come from my years of experience in the fitness industry. It is my hope that people will use health and fitness to ignite their own personal growth.

Setting a goal requires inspiration, an initial thought or slight change in perspective that triggers the desire for personal improvement. Motivation through inspiration is a simple concept that holds true for any scenario in life. Inspiration provides a purpose for action. This, in turn sustains the motivation and discipline required to execute a course of action, thereby resulting in achievement of the goal.

The Performance Continuum Paradigm© assumes that growth and increasingly higher performance is a constant process that also includes planning and awareness. It provides a philosophical basis for people to strategically move forward in life by using physical health as the vehicle for success. For one to become truly successful in the achievement of their goals, it is absolutely crucial that you engage in some self-reflection first. Then make your goals tangible by constructing a realistic but flexible action plan with timelines. Finally, keep yourself accountable for carrying out the plan while occasionally revisiting and restructuring it.

Within The Performance Continuum Paradigm©, individual lives are seen to be composed of five life components; Physical, Mental, Emotional, Financial and Spiritual. In the diagram above, they form the *Central Pyramid.* These components are part of the life of every individual and they all influence each other.

PHYSICAL This component relates to your physical health and performance, and essentially forms the foundation. If you have your physical health, are exercising regularly and have a healthy diet, you will feel more energetic, rest better, be more confident, and have a better sense of self overall.

MENTAL This component is directly influenced by the foundation—your physical health. Being health-conscious and active can increase mental clarity and stability. It also reduces unhealthy stress levels in your life.

EMOTIONAL Your emotional awareness and your ability to have positive and effective relationships with others are significantly affected by your physical and mental strength. Emotional strength promotes confidence and self-awareness.

FINANCIAL In today's society, financial obligations are a part of everyone's life. Financial stability and professional aspirations are achieved through being clear about what you want and need to do to get them. If you are consistently focused on improving who you are as a person, your ability to become more financially stable is increased.

SPIRITUAL While spiritual strength and awareness is unique to the individual, it invariably allows people to be more connected not only with themselves and as well as with others. Through self-development we increase our sense of self, sharpen our awareness of what we stand for, and what our true purpose is in life, career, relationships, and the world.

The *Central Pyramid* is heavily influenced by the Internal and External Factors that impact your decision-making process. They may be positive, like internalized core values you've learned growing up. They may be negative, as when the media experts tell you what the ideal body should look like. The key to dealing with these Internal and External Factors is being aware that they are, in fact, present, and that they impact everyone.

Being clear on what you want and what you stand for will help you maintain your core values. However it is also important to have safeguards in place to ensure that you stay within the boundaries you have established for yourself. These could include a support system of friends and/or family that assist with keeping you on track towards your goals. Sharing your goals with those who support you can be a great way to enhance your rate of success.

The Performance Continuum Paradigm© is a practical model of healthy living that is put into practice using a system that provides a continuously changing focus and re-establishment of goals every 90 days to ensure both progression and variety. Its four stages are called the 4 C's, which are characterized by a focus on Core, Cardiovascular Endurance, Consumption and Challenge.

CORE

When starting any program, establishing balanced Core Strength (physical) and Core Values (mental) are essential to a strong foundation.

CARDIOVASCULAR

The next step is to build up your cardiovascular endurance and also your mental resilience. Using calories effectively not only aids in decreasing the risk of heart disease and enhancing physical performance, but also indirectly affects your mental stamina, clarity and focus.

CONSUMPTION

Everything you take in both physically and mentally has an effect on you. How your body metabolizes food, how your mind makes decisions, and the state of your overall health are all affected. Hydration and nutrition are key factors in maintaining and maximizing a healthy lifestyle. Equally important are what you read, what you watch on TV, your relationships, and what you choose to think and talk about. All can have positive or negative effects on your goals.

CHALLENGE

The final stage in this progression is also the beginning of a brand new cycle. Like any new stimulus in life (whether physical or mental), your body and mind must adapt to it. This is why typically we see great results in the beginning of a workout routine, new job, new relationships, etc. However as this stimulus becomes more and more predictable, changes stop occurring. We find our once new and exciting stimulus becoming monotonous and just another task to complete. Research supports the positive effects of purposeful and positive change to promote goal-oriented results. If you do not challenge yourself in life you become stagnant. What's *your* next challenge?

THE FOUR PHASES OF BECOMING FIT

Over the next four chapters, I'm going to take you through four of the phases your mind will go through as you incorporate new and healthy habits into your lifestyle on your way to awakening your Inner Athlete.

First is the ***Dreamer Phase.*** A couple of weeks into the process of becoming fit, you are going to start looking at people who've already achieved your goal and you may want to be like them. At the same time your mind is going to start playing tricks on you. The first thing that will strike you is the realization that it's going to take some hard work to achieve this goal. That's the kind of opening that the pessimistic part of your nature just loves. So don't be surprised if you start coming up with all kinds of reasons why your plans are not going to work.

Don't ever discount the power of pessimism. It's what stops 95% of people who start fitness programs from carrying on until they find their "inner athlete". We are going to come up with a strategy to beat that pessimism.

Next is the **Doer Phase**. People in this phase are putting in the time and effort but may have unrealistic expectations about the time it takes to achieve their goals. So they keep trying—harder and harder. Alternatively, they may think their efforts are effective, when in fact they may be the exact opposite.

As you might expect, this can lead to discouragement or even physical injury. However, if you realize you are in this phase, you can consciously manage your expectations and slow yourself down. We'll meet a few of the people I've worked with whose stories will provide you with insight into the experiences they had while going through this phase.

Of course sooner or later you are bound to come to the **Plateau Phase.** Your initial resolve and drive have leveled off. You are still doing the exercises but mentally you're no longer with the program. This is another critical time. Mental monotony can lead to physical flat lining. You will probably need a refresher course in the holistic and lifestyle aspects of your program—a mental booster shot. Without it you'll likely find that your attitude starts holding you back. This has the possibility of promoting injury, weight gain, mood swings, sleepless nights and other physiological abnormalities. This will be the time for a complete change in stimulus—some new mental exercises and workout suggestions to inspire you to push to a new level of physical and mental challenge.

This inspiration will eventually lead to the **Breakthrough Phase.** When you break through, then you are fully with the program. You will understand—deep within your soul—

that while life is full of plateaus, you can work strategically to minimize the length of time you'll spend on any of them. You'll become self-reflective and strive to go in the direction of challenge and eliminate your fears. Variety will become something you value highly and purposefully work into your life plan.

Becoming mentally and physically fit is one of the most important and rewarding challenges that you will ever undertake. Each of these four phases has rewards and drawbacks. I believe that by recognizing the phases as you go through them, you will be better prepared to successfully work through to the conclusion of the program.

It will be your time of awakening.

Fit Tip

Now that you have a framework to explore where you currently are in your life, try to determine what factors may be influencing you, and how you can strategically approach goal attainment, I would like for you to start creating your action plan. We will start with getting things out of your mind and onto paper.

When you register on-line you receive access to one month of on-line coaching from me personally and access to my special fitness and lifestyle tools, including the Life Strategy Worksheet mentioned in this chapter. You can register anytime by visiting *www.IAmBishop. com/ThinkFactor.*

Chapter Four

The Dreamer Phase

Daydreaming about your future achievements can be very powerful. But it can also be extremely unproductive if you don't take action to make your dreams come true.

The Dreamer Phase is characterized by encouraging thoughts and a real desire to be better, feel better and be healthier. The length of time people remain at this stage is dependent on many factors, including their environment, upbringing, support system, and financial capability. Although these factors may vary, the ability to succeed is always present if they want it enough.

Here are three stories that illustrate what I mean…

JUDY'S JOURNEY

When it came to exercise, Judy was a novice. I started working with her a year ago when she came to me in desperation. She was never a "thin" person and was ok with that, but she found herself beginning to gain more weight than she wanted to.

During our health consultation she told me about her sense of frustration with how her image had more recently taken a turn for the worse. It seemed to stem from certain aspects of her childhood.

Physical exercise was never really a part of Judy's life as she was growing up. Her parents were overweight and her siblings also had weight problems. It occurred to me that Judy—quite unconsciously—felt destined to continue that cycle. It was all she knew.

Judy is only in her late twenties and still has lots of time to turn things around. She wanted to break her unhealthy habits so that her children (ages two and four) would grow up and follow a healthier lifestyle than the one she grew up with.

Judy told me that when she and her husband met, they weren't exactly skinny but they definitely weren't where they both are today—each of them is at least 50 pounds overweight.

Psychologically, this fact was perhaps the biggest challenge Judy had to overcome. Just the thought of having to lose all that weight would be discouraging to anyone. Starting to exercise and get into a healthier routine seemed so daunting that she just didn't know where to start. What was worse, she didn't think it would do any good to try.

Of course there were moments of inspiration, moments of having had enough of being a couch potato. Sometimes that was enough to encourage Judy to get outside for walks or invest in a gym membership. But these moments where so short lived that she could never build up enough momentum to keep herself going longer than a couple of weeks. Then it was back to old habits and new pounds.

As Judy's personal coach and trainer, my job was as much psychological as it was physical. There really was no reason for her to be so overweight, and she was young enough and healthy enough that losing the extra pounds was certainly possible. The real question was whether she could maintain the momentum long enough to achieve it.

It was slow going at first, but as Judy began to make progress one step at a time, she started to believe in herself. During our sessions she would tell me about her past attempts to lose weight by exercising every week. She would tune in to one or more of the reality TV weight loss programs.. These programs would uplift her at times and present her with many things that she could relate to. Sometimes she felt as though a particular weight loss participant was in the exact same predicament as she was. She would tell herself that tomorrow would be different. Tomorrow she would get up early and invest in her health. Tomorrow morning she would start doing some form of exercise. Tomorrow afternoon she would go grocery shopping and buy all the right things and prepare her meals for work in advance. Of course "tomorrow" never seemed to come.

The pattern was always the same. For a day or two Judy would get excited and decide to start something. However before she could really begin, her family responsibilities, the indifference of those around her, and the comfort of the old day-to-day routine would combine to gently but firmly push her off track. As the attempts and failures added up, she became increasingly frustrated and stressed. Out of desperation she ended up using those two powerful negatives—junk food and TV—to distract her from what she had vowed to do.

Summertime had become particularly difficult for Judy. As the weather became warmer, there were many things she wished she could do. She would see active people head to the streets jogging and cycling. They made it look easy.

"Why can't I do that"? she said to herself. "Why can't I enjoy exercising outdoors"? It was as if she was trying to do a completely foreign activity.

After months of pondering, dreaming, and talking herself into it, one day she finally worked up the courage and jogged down the sidewalk. Within a couple of minutes she had to stop, gasping for breath. It was exhausting. She felt nothing but pain and the embarrassment of thinking that everyone was watching her and judging her performance. So what did she do? She retreated back inside the house, where she was comfortable, and spent the rest of the afternoon on the couch watching others do what she wanted to do.

After months of similar attempts—all of which ended up with her back in her comfort zone in front of the TV—Judy came to a realization. The principal reason for her lack of consistency and inability to follow through with her self-taught health and fitness program was that she lacked a support system that would help her stay with her goal for more than a day or two. If Judy really wanted to successfully achieve her twin goals of losing weight and becoming more active, she needed the continual support, encouragement and persistence of caring people around her—people who would continually work with her and hold her accountable.

In more than 90 percent of the cases I've encountered, lack of adequate encouragement and support is what prevents people from getting the momentum they need to stay with their fitness programs and meet their goals. Judy's dream was to end the cycle of unhealthy living and weight gain that her family was so accustomed to. She wanted to develop the drive and determination that would allow her to be the role model for her kids and her family. But she had to put a support group in place to make that dream come true.

TOM'S JOURNEY

Tom is the enthusiastic Type A business executive who dives into things at full speed without looking back.

As a fitness professional, in many ways, working with Tom provides me with a refreshing change. He buys into the program plan, understands the benefits and demands the same commitment to his exercise regimen as he does from his career.

Tom grew up an avid athlete, playing a variety of sports throughout high school and college. Now, 42 years old, having spent many years building a successful career, he came to me with the desire to get back physically to where he used to be. He had added some unwanted fat around his waist, was subject to nagging knee and back pain, and was not content with his current health and fitness condition.

"I used to be so fit," was how he put it.

Tom and I got to know each other quickly within our first month. He began by sharing his memories of his college football days—the game-winning touchdowns and how people were awed at his ability. Pushing modesty to the side at times, he liked to stress just how "fit and athletic" he was at that time in his life.

Even though Tom was undeniably an accomplished athlete—perhaps even an elite athlete in his younger days— he was at the Dreamer Phase at this stage in his life. When it came to health and fitness, he tended to hang onto memories. When speaking of his goals, he would identify with current sports stars.

Now don't get me wrong. There is nothing wrong with identifying with athletes, past or present. The problem in Tom's case is that he was what I consider a "weekend warrior" who would often decide at the last minute, to run a marathon, or sign up for an adventure race. Only later did he realize he would have to get up at 6:00 am the next Saturday to take part in a grueling three-day event without having done any physical preparation.

Because of that, I soon discovered that his previous training methods—or lack of training—had taken a toll on his body. My first task, therefore, was to convince him to take a few steps back in order to get into the kind of shape that would prepare him to move forward safely and effectively.

Tom's dream is be as youthful, lean, fast and powerful as he so vividly remembers himself being. His goals are to get back to playing hockey recreationally and to begin competing in running events and adventure races again without the added pain.

He realized that he had some limitations. His history of not preparing for strenuous activities resulted in a number of injuries that had not healed properly. But also, he now realized that he must work at it consistently.

I had no doubt that he would do it.

Kim's Journey

"I grew up a tomboy and was very athletic," said Kim, who was offered a scholarship for basketball and volleyball by University of Michigan. She declined because at that time she was married and wanted to have a family. "I was on every starting team in high school, whether it was volleyball, basketball, or track-and-field."

However, after giving birth to her first child at 20, her activity level dropped off dramatically. "I never really had an interest in fitness per se," she said. "I had an interest in team sports. I never really paid much attention to diet and after my daughter started going to daycare I got into the habit of buying whatever was quick and convenient."

After Kim had her second child, she found that she had completely lost her drive for an active lifestyle. "At that point I did nothing but lots of eating."

With the demands of family life, Kim found that her time was not always her own. Because she never really had an interest in fitness, she never got back into team sports and her diet took a turn towards "convenient eating" as opposed to healthy eating.

Meanwhile, as an accomplished singer/song writer, Kim had aspirations of taking her singing career to the next level. "I had the opportunity to perform at Summer Jam, which at the time was a really big deal," she said. "This scared me in a way because I felt I needed to do something about how I looked. I pushed myself to get into the gym so I could look my best. Because I had no idea how to workout or what to do, I just ran on the treadmill almost every day for a month and dropped over 10 lbs". After performing at Summer Jam, she went right back to her inactive lifestyle.

However, Kim had learned that it was possible to get back into shape if she could summon up the motivation and the drive to make it a priority. Not only did she get a glimpse of how prioritizing regular exercise into your routine actually works, but during her month of commitment to exercise, she also became more confident and focused.

At this stage in her life, the biggest obstacle for Kim was the lack of a plan that was realistic in terms of family and career demands. She needed a plan that was interest-driven, so it would be something she would set as a personal priority. While consulting with Kim it became apparent that she needed assistance to create a plan that tapped into her love for the sources of true inspiration in her life—her family, team sports and her rising singing career.

With that in mind, we began her fitness journey.

Whether you are someone who is brand new to fitness, or a person who often thinks about getting fit and envies those who seem to make it happen so easily; there is always a way for you to succeed. It all begins with a dream.

The Dreamer Phase is where you start the process of knowing and unleashing your inner-athlete. I use the term inner-athlete to describe the drive that inspires you. It's a spark that is different for every individual. It may be a memorable childhood activity that still motivates you. It may be a sport that you still love, a life-changing event like the birth of a child, travel to a new country, a career change, even a tragedy. Everyone has it. If you haven't yet identified the spark that drives your inner-athlete— look for it! Start by remembering the things that have purpose and meaning to you. The more important that purpose is, the more successful you will become at unleashing your inner-athlete to achieve the lifestyle and fitness goals you want.

Before you read on, take ten minutes to brainstorm and write down any sources of inspiration that come to you. There is no wrong way to go about this. The main purpose is to get you thinking about what motivates you to take action. Some questions to consider:

- ✓ What past activities can you recall that excited and that inspire you?

- ✓ What are some current activities that you enjoy and inspire you?

- ✓ What activities and experiences do you want to try out, incorporate or accomplish in the future?

Fit Tip

Start with a dream and then translate it to an action plan. The first step is to write down your thoughts. Take ten minutes to do a lifestyle check. Here's how...

On a piece of paper or on your computer, create two columns.

Label the left column Healthy Lifestyle and the right one Unhealthy Lifestyle.

Reflect on the past month, listing things like items you have purchased, choices you have made, things you have done, etc. under the appropriate heading.

Then spend the next month doing the things you've listed in the Healthy Lifestyle column and avoiding things in the Unhealthy Lifestyle column.

As you go through the month, you'll notice it becomes easier to do the healthy things while avoiding the unhealthy ones. This is an easy way to start creating momentum towards the fulfillment of your own dreams.

What follows is a general Fitness Evaluation for you to complete in order to identify your current fitness level. It is important to know where you are heading as well as where you are starting from. This Fitness Evaluation will also allow you to set some tangible benchmarks to achieve in your new fitness journey.

Based on your fitness evaluation score, you will begin with one of three fitness programs provided in the next chapter. The program you begin with will be determined by your current fitness level and abilities. Everyone has a starting point and these three programs are applicable—whether you are a novice just starting out or someone who needs to stop dreaming and kick-start their current exercise routine.

These programs are designed for convenience, with minimal equipment necessary. You can complete most of the exercises in the comfort of your own home, without having to go to a gym. It's a great way to make your game plan excuse-proof! Let's get started now with your fitness evaluation.

BODY COMPOSITION

I suggest that you schedule an appointment to have your body composition tested by a personal trainer. However, if you do not have access to one, you should at least record your body weight and girth measurements (as shown on the Fitness Evaluation Table—page 53) so that you have a benchmark to start from.

12-MINUTE-RUN TEST

Provided you have no knee or joint problems that prevent you from running, I recommend the 12-minute-run test for a good benchmark of your cardiovascular endurance. For this test, choose a block in your neighborhood, the circumference of a park, or even a track, that is convenient for you and also relatively flat.

If you have a heart rate monitor, this will be beneficial to get an idea of your "One Minute Heart Rate Recovery" at the end of the 12-minute-run. This is basically a measurement of how fast your heart rate drops from its maximum measurement (at the end of the test) in one minute. You can record this in the Fitness Evaluation Table within the 12-minute-run section by simply subtracting your ending heart rate (at 12 minutes) from your heart rate reading at 13 minutes. As you continue with a regular fitness program that involves cardiovascular conditioning, you will notice during a retest that your "One Minute Heart Rate Recovery" shows a larger drop (in beats/minute) in the one-minute time frame than the previous test. This is a sign of cardiovascular improvement. Essentially your body shows that it is more capable of a faster recovery, therefore better able to deliver oxygenated blood to the working muscles.

As you start this test, try to run the entire 12 minutes; if you can't make the full 12 minutes, take note of where you had to stop and continue to power walk until you are able to run again. The idea is to try to cover as much distance (as many rounds of the block) as you can in the 12-minute time frame, so the faster you go the more distance you will cover. If you do this on a track, you will know that every lap is 400 meters and you can calculate your exact distance at the end of the test. If you are using a block in your neighborhood try to still complete as many laps as you can. Be sure you take note of where you stop at the end of the 12 minutes by using a landmark like light post or fire hydrant. The next time you do the 12-minute-run test, your distance will surpass your previous stopping point landmark.

PUSH-UP TEST

For this exercise you will perform as many push-ups as you can with good form. If you can only do push-ups from your knees, no problem—start there. If you can do some push ups from your feet then start there. Take note of when you have to go to your knees to complete the test. If you can only complete a few full push-ups, again that is no problem. Each time you do this test you will see an improvement in the number of quality reps you can accomplish. To ensure you are getting a full range of motion on each rep use a towel rolled up and placed underneath the chest as a marker so that each time your chest touches it you can count that as one rep.

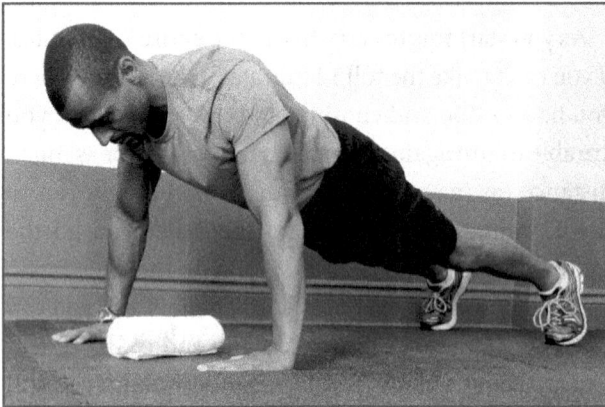

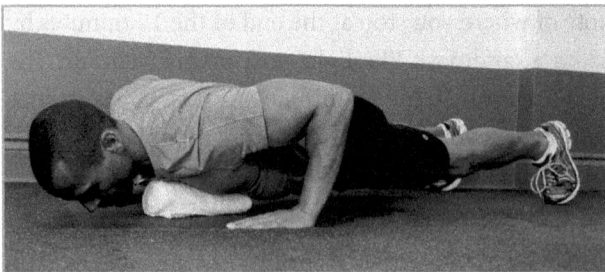

- ❏ Start with chest directly over your hands and hands slightly wider than shoulder width

- ❏ From the knees or feet lower your body so that your chest touches the towel

- ❏ Exhale and push back up until your arms are fully extended

- ❏ Repeat for as many reps as you can and record the reps from knees and/or feet

TIP: keep your core tight and posture straight throughout the movement. Hips should be in line with shoulders as shown.

WALL SIT TEST

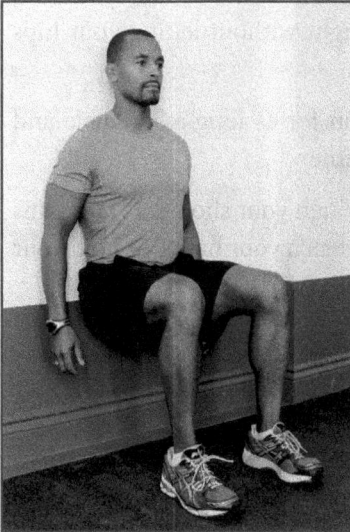

- ❏ Start with your back against a wall, posture straight and knees at 90 degrees

- ❏ Keep your weight on your heels, and arms relaxed at your side

- ❏ Hold this position for as long as you can and record how long you held it

ABDOMINAL PLANK TEST

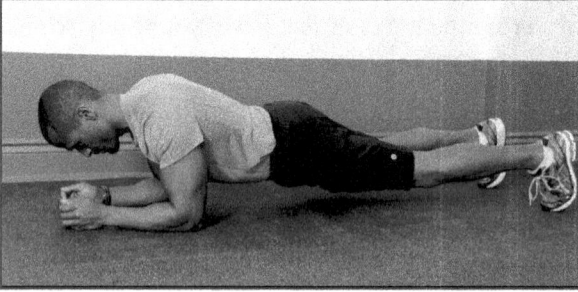

❏ Position yourself on your forearms and toes with core tight and posture straight

❏ Shoulder joints should remain directly above the elbow joints

❏ Draw belly button in towards the spine and keep your core tight without letting your hips drop

❏ Hold this position for as long as possible and record the final time

TIP: to stay relaxed through your shoulders and arms during the test, do not clench your hands or hold your breath.

FITNESS EVALUATION TABLE

QUARTERLY FITNESS EVALUATION	Q1	Q2	Q3	Q4
Body Composition (lbs)				
Scale Weight				
Lean Weight				
Fat Weight				
Body Fat %				
*may be completed at a fitness center				
Girth Measurements (cm)				
Waist				
Mid Thigh				
Bust/Chest				
Flexed Arm				
*measuring tape required				
Cardiovascular Endurance				
12 Min Block Run (# of blocks)				
*use landmark for end of 12 min				
Muscular Endurance				
Pushups (maximum number)				
*record # from feet and/or # from knees				
Wall Sit (min)				
Abdominal Plank (min)				

Chapter Five

THE DOER PHASE

Action is perhaps the single most important force in promoting change, whether positive or negative. Without it we remain stagnant.

Have you ever really considered what you were going to accomplish in your day—how you would get up early, go for a run, and have a balanced breakfast, followed by a fulfilling day of accomplishment at work?

Transitioning from The Dreamer to The Doer phase essentially involves taking these thoughts and dreams and making them real. Then you actually start to do what you envision rather than just think about it.

This phase has its advantages and disadvantages. People in this stage could be transitioning from The Dreamer phase and progressing towards achieving their goals. Conversely, they could be people with unrealistic expectations, who have been stuck in The Doer phase for some time. They have become discouraged and unable to move forward with a clear focus because they've been taking ineffective action.

JUDY'S JOURNEY

Judy was ready. It had been too long. There had been too many years of poor lifestyle choices. There had been too much time spent dreaming about a healthy life and a healthy weight; but too little time spent doing something about it. Judy had finally made the decision to put her thoughts into action and commit to a fitness routine.

As I listened to her describe the struggle she has been in for years, and the trend toward obesity that has plagued her family, I could tell right away that something had inspired her, something had brought her to a state of action. She couldn't tolerate her current situation anymore. She wanted change so much that she was finally willing to put it all on the line. This is my ideal client to work with—someone who is committed to the process and truly wants to change.

However, after a few sessions in the gym with Judy, I found myself changing my initial thoughts. Judy was going to have difficulty with the effort required to achieve what she wanted. Although losing about 50 pounds was realistic over time, during her exercise sessions, Judy was not really prepared to focus, or to put in the kind of effort needed to be successful.

There is a simple saying: "If your mind is not in it, you cannot win it". This applies to every situation I have ever come across. My concern was that Judy's lack of focus and commitment would increase the time required to achieve significant results to the point where it would hinder her chance of success.

In Judy's mind, the fact that she had started a regular fitness program meant she should immediately see great results. This attitude will inevitably result in discouragement and, in the worst case, failure to achieve ones goals.

There was a definite disconnect between what I was asking of Judy and what she was actually doing. She had seemed so ready, driven, and eager to get into a fitness program when I first consulted with her. What was going wrong?

I didn't realize it at first, but in her mind, Judy had actually achieved her initial goal—to make a commitment to a regular exercise routine. She had done this by physically coming to the gym and also by making a financial commitment to improve her health. Now I had to coach her to the next step—making this commitment effective by becoming mentally committed to the process as much as to the dream.

People sometimes have a dream or idea of exactly what they want, but fall short once they are placed in a position to achieve it. In my experience, much of this stems from a false belief that by committing time or money, they have, in fact, done what is required. They forget that they have not made the behavioral changes that are required to achieve their goal.

Often, they will remain within their comfort zone; keeping the wall up and unconsciously preventing or delaying themselves from moving forward. This usually leads to discouragement—the feeling that they have been putting in their time but haven't experienced the results they expected. It was apparent Judy's approach to her new commitment was, in fact, holding her back.

As I get to know clients I will occasionally introduce them to new activities to help me find out what makes them tick. I was determined to see what made Judy tick. The fun part of this is that quite often they do not even know themselves what gets them excited.

It was the end of Week Two. After much discussion and coaching on the amount of effort required to progressively see results, I decided Judy needed something completely different. That's when we put on the boxing gloves.

I had no idea she could hit so hard! She was a completely different person behind those gloves! She had never experienced boxing before, nor imagined herself doing it, but something within her was very focused, confident and powerful. Wow—did that ever unleash her inner athlete! With Judy, boxing seemed to be (pardon the pun) bang on.

Not only did she put tremendous effort into the boxing drills, but the pent-up anger and stress she released during the activity also proved to be very therapeutic for her. After we introduced boxing and incorporated more self-defense training into her program; Judy brought greater effort to each session which elevated and transferred to other exercises— even ones she did not like. She became competitive within herself; a quality that is necessary to excel and move forward in The Doer phase.

Tom's Journey

The weekend after our initial meeting, Tom ran about 40 kilometers. The combination of not running for years, as well as his previous history of knee injuries and back issues, left him feeling crippled as a result. It was definitely not the ideal start for this all-or-nothing Doer, but he was focused on getting to his goal of feeling athletic again without the pain.

Tom was highly motivated from the start. But, if unchecked, his Type A personality and apparent need for control could damage his ability to succeed. He definitely required guidance on how to be effective with his fitness program so that he didn't fall into the trap of remaining in The Doer phase, thereby becoming frustrated because his over-activity got in the way of achieving his goals.

Initially the need for him to moderate his training volume and intensity was difficult for him to accept. I had to frequently tell him to slow-down and focus on the basics first, I also had to prescribe very specific homework for him to do. For Tom, the key to progress was for him to understand that this approach would get him to his ultimate goals without further damaging his body.

Once he understood this, Tom's natural athleticism and mental drive became purposely focused, which was a great foundation for his ultimate success. I found his progress and consistency to be particularly helpful. His joint stabilizers became stronger, his core strength more balanced, and his entire neuromuscular system began to respond effectively. It was time for us to step up his program before he became bored with the routine.

During the warm up for a session one afternoon, Tom didn't seem like himself. He was very withdrawn. Apparently a huge deal at work had fallen through—one that he was almost sure he had closed. We discussed it for a while but I soon came to the realization that talking about it was doing more harm than good. Tom did not like to dwell on what wasn't working. He preferred to move on to the next situation—one over which he had some control.

This was the perfect time to get Tom looking forward. To pique his interest, I began to make suggestions that he enter some upcoming events. He is a very competitive person and it didn't take much to get a complete attention shift. He became very alert, animated, and excited. Once again illustrating how a complete physiological change can be initiated by a shift in one's mindset. That's why controlling your mindset can be so powerful.

Together we talked about what interests him and what I thought would be suitable for him while avoiding further injury. Tom's nagging injuries came from years of repetitive exercise—typically running without proper training.

I knew Tom loved activities like hiking and mountain biking—this was a good thing as it allowed me to suggest a multi-sport event that would be easier on his joints. We decided on a competition that is a three-day event involving trail running, hiking, paddling, mountain biking, and navigation. It is also a destination event that takes place in Colorado and covers nearly 300 kilometres with varied terrain and elevations. We had almost a full year to prepare for it.

I also suggested some "mini-events" over the next year to prepare Tom for this competition. Part of this strategy was to ensure that Tom would focus on both the short and long-term goals while continuing to experience the excitement of meeting a challenge for which he needed to train effectively. We agreed that he would enter three races leading up to this event in Colorado—a half-marathon, a mountain biking endurance race and a smaller multi-sport race that involved a 21 km run, 80 km bike, and 40 km kayak segments. By training for three modes of activity, we also reduced the wear and tear that a single distance sport would have on Tom's muscles and joints. He became focused, excited and ready to live out the plan.

KIM'S JOURNEY

All Kim needed was to get going—so we did. From the start, the goal was to bring the idea of team sports back into her routine. We began one-on-one sessions twice a week. She also signed up for an athletic conditioning class every Saturday. This was enough to generate the momentum and consistency that empowered her to regain control of her lifestyle. Volleyball had been Kim's passion from an early age so I began to incorporate volleyball drills and sport-specific training into her sessions.

The outcome was amazing.

After just a month of working with Kim, the change in her mental focus, physical strength and overall fitness level were remarkable. The momentum had been created—she was more focused with her career direction and family life, and after each training session she would be closer to her goals. After a few months, Kim enrolled in a recreational volleyball league and loved every minute of it. We continued to work on her jumping, agility, speed, and hand-eye coordination so that she would continue to improve her game and out-perform others on the volleyball court.

My approach to helping Kim achieve her goals was to use multi-joint or compound movements for her exercises. This involves working more than one muscle and moving more than one joint at a time. Often traditional exercise routines, which use the concept of muscle isolation, doing the same exercises and routines over and over again, can bore people.

The benefit of the multi-joint/compound movement approach is that it not only increases the mental and neurological involvement (i.e., preventing boredom and maximizing performance) but also elevates metabolism and cardiovascular improvement—training the body as a whole.

This kind of interest-driven program also allows participants to remain focused on that which they are passionate about. It brings purpose to their training routine which then crosses over to their activities, sports and life in general. Additionally, as a result of the strength and cardiovascular conditioning, they are also able to achieve their underlying goals of weight loss and toning.

At this point, Kim also needed more structured assistance with her nutrition. With her new focus on exercise, she was naturally more conscious of what she was eating. However, she still needed more direction on how nutrition could help her maximize her success. As with all my clients, I began by having Kim log her daily food and fluid intake so I could provide her with some direction. This would also hold her accountable for what she was eating. The best way to succeed in anything is by setting small goals and achieving them daily. This would help her build confidence, self-esteem, and help habituate the positive changes that she is looking for.

To help Kim even more, we set some concrete goals to be attained by specific dates—ones that were now very important to her. Kim had recently been notified that she had been nominated for a Juno Award. She was extremely excited but also nervous. She wanted to look and feel her best. After doing her second fitness evaluation and seeing significant results, we changed the stimulus to ensure Kim moved to the next level to achieve her new goals by the day of the Juno Awards presentation. The Junos proved to be a perfect date to work towards. We marshaled Kim's nervous and excited energy to fuel a new exercise routine that had her working out six days a week.

THE COMMON THREAD

It is human nature to do what inspires you. Quite often it is impossible to resist. When you are inspired, your priorities centre on your source of inspiration. This results in a shift in perspective and creates an inner drive that motivates you. The unfortunate part is that not everyone is aware of what inspires them, or they forget to keep looking for inspiration. When you lose your sense of play and curiosity you are basically on autopilot, letting life live you instead of you living life.

The above stories illustrate how different types of people have rediscovered something that inspires them. This gets them moving and excited about life and achieving their goals. For Judy, it was a complete shift in perspective. Using boxing—

which she had never done before—stimulated her mind and body. This enabled her to add effort to her fitness routine. In turn she began to feel powerful and increasingly confident. Naturally results started to come her way.

Tom needed to be in control and operating on extremes. His mindset was difficult to change. However, once he had a program that combined an approach that let him circumvent injury, and have a clear vision of how he could become an athlete again—he had purpose and direction.

The common thread with people in The Doer phase is momentum—taking one step forward and exploring activities or perspectives that create awareness and new ways of doing. As observed in these three examples, the initial motivation of doing things differently led to new results. Instead of just dreaming and being frustrated with what they were not; Judy, Tom, and Kim now had a vision of what they could be.

Fit Tip

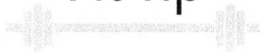

NOW YOU ARE READY TO START!

With your Fitness Evaluation completed, you know your current fitness level. Based on your results, choose the program in the next chapter which will be most suitable for you to begin your fitness routine.

Chapter Six

THE STARTER PROGRAMS

MEDICAL DISCLAIMER

All information in this book is presented for educational purposes only. This general information is not intended to diagnose any medical condition or to replace your healthcare professional.

Always consult your physician before beginning any exercise program. Most individuals can safely participate in light to moderate physical activity programs.

If you have any injury, disease, disability or other concern about starting an exercise program, consult your healthcare provider first.

WHEN TO CONTACT YOUR PHYSICIAN

Howerver, if you experience any symptoms of weakness, unsteadiness, light-headed-ness or dizziness, chest pain or pressure, nausea, or shortness of breath.

Mild soreness after exercise may be experienced after beginning a new exercise. Contact your physician if the soreness does not improve after 2-3 days.

STARTER PROGRAM

LEVEL ONE *(Novice/Beginner)*

REQUIREMENTS:

- Less than 12 minutes of continuous jogging
- Less than 15 Push Ups from the knees
- Less than 1 minute on the Abdominal Plank
- Less than 1 minute on the Wall Sit

PROGRAM DETAILS:

- Program Length: 6 weeks
- Workout Duration: 25-30 minutes per workout
- Frequency: 2 days per week
- Result: Tone your body without leaving the house!

TOOLS REQUIRED:

- Hand towel
- 2 Chairs
- 2 Small hand weights
- 1 Broomstick

WARM-UP

5 – 10 minutes—skipping, jogging, cycling

COMPLETE 2 SETS

OF THIS 5 EXERCISE SEQUENCE

GLIDING REVERSE LUNGE

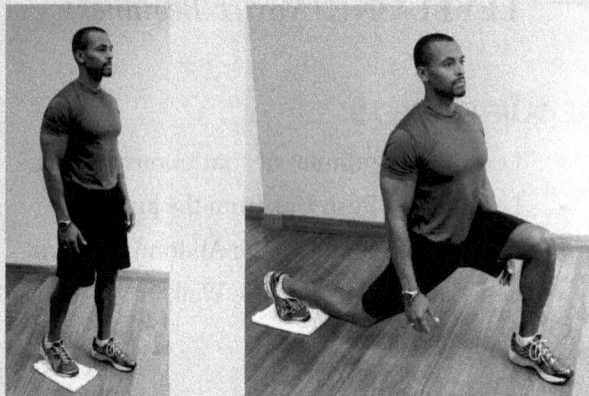

- To be completed on hardwood or tile floor
- Start with one foot on towel and opposite foot on floor
- Slide rear foot backwards
- Push off front heel and return to starting position
- Complete 10 -15 repetitions per leg
- **TIP:** try not to pull with rear foot and keep pressure on front heel throughout.

CHAIR PUSH UP

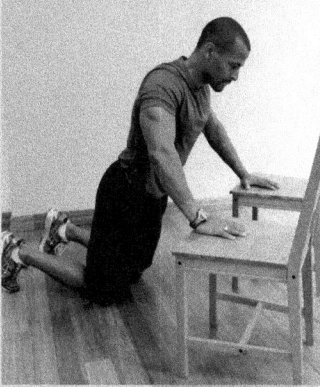

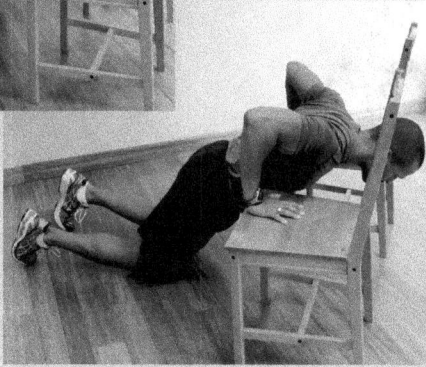

- Position two stable chairs further than shoulder width apart
- With one hand on each chair in a kneeling position descend between chairs
- Exhale and push yourself back up to start position
- Complete 15 repetitions
- **TIP**: to increase difficulty, try from a standing position. Ensure you keep your core engaged throughout the exercise.

REVERSE FLY

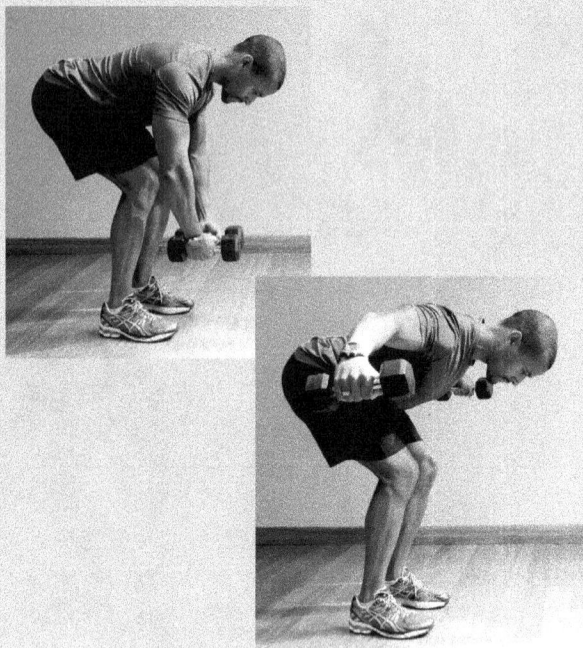

- Holding hand weights, bend parallel to ground with palms facing inward

- Elbows in a fixed but slightly bent position, raise arms towards ceiling

- Slowly return arms back to starting position.

- Complete 15 repetitions

- **TIP:** keep head neutral and do not elevate shoulders towards your ears

OVERHEAD POSTURAL SQUAT

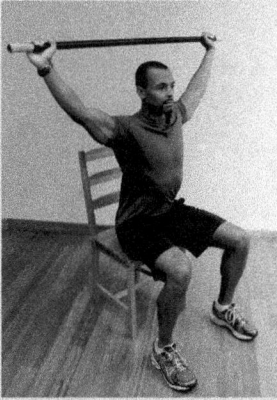

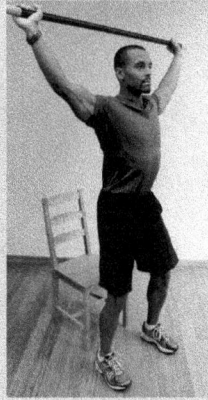

- Stand in front of a chair with feet slightly wider than shoulder width

- Hold broomstick in wide grip position with arms straight and far back

- Slowly lower your body down to chair by sinking hips back and down

- From chair, push through heels driving back up to start position

- Complete 10-15 repetitions

- **TIP:** Goal is to keep broomstick in line with spine while coming out of squat position without momentum or forward lean

GLIDING ABDOMINAL TUCK

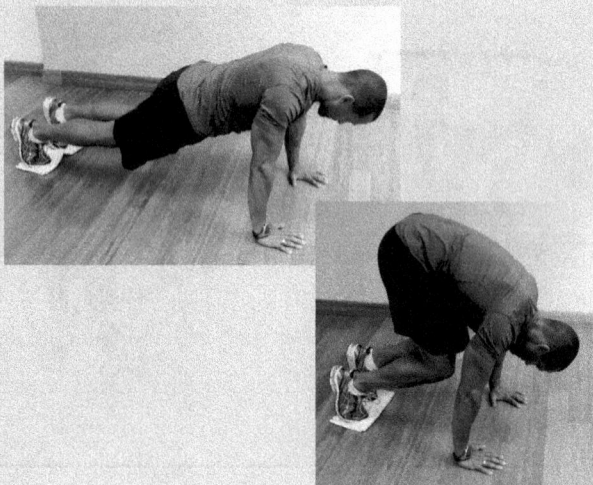

- Place hands on floor, shoulder width apart and feet on towel

- Pulling from the waist, glide the feet towards your hands while hips elevate

- Extend back out to starting position

- Complete 15 repetitions (if you can't complete repetitions, just hold the 1st position)

- To increase difficulty, try with straight knees

- **TIP:** Ensure shoulders are directly above your hands throughout the exercise

STARTER PROGRAM

LEVEL TWO *(Beginner/Intermediate)*

REQUIREMENTS:

- Complete 12 minutes of continuous jogging
- More than 15 push ups from the knees or 5 push ups from the feet
- More than 1 minute on the abdominal plank
- More than 1 minute on the wall sit

PROGRAM DETAILS:

- Program Length: 6 weeks
- Workout Duration: 25 - 30 minutes per workout, minimal rest between exercises
- Frequency: 3 days per week

TOOLS REQUIRED:

- Resistance Band (medium tension)
- Medicine Ball

WARM-UP

5 – 10 minutes—skipping, jogging, cycling

COMPLETE 2 - 3 SETS
OF THIS 5 EXERCISE SEQUENCE

☑ Increase intensity by adding 1-2 minutes of skipping at the end of each 5 exercise sequence

REVERSE LUNGE – SHOULDER PRESS

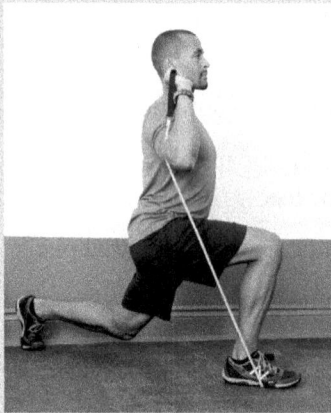

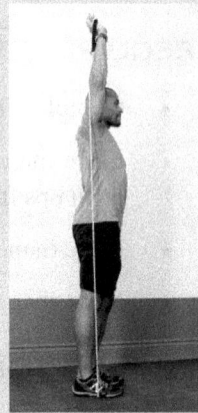

- Anchor resistance band under one foot to desired tension
- Hold handle at shoulder height, step backwards into lunge position
- Come up out of lunge while pressing resistance up
- Complete 15 repetitions per side
- **TIP:** Always emphasize your weight through your front heel

MED-BALL SQUAT THRUST

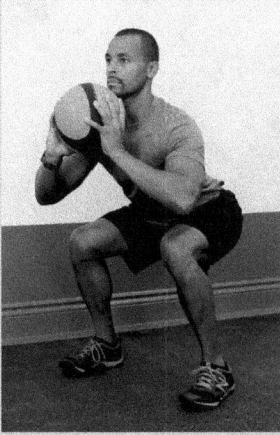

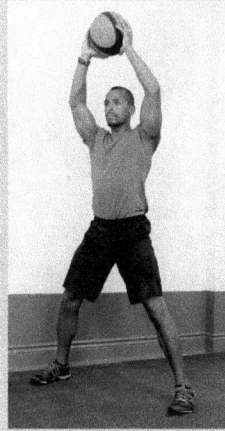

- Hold med-ball in both hands at chest level while in squat position
- Quickly jump out of squat into a wide foot position while pressing med-ball overhead
- Drop back into starting position absorbing your landing to 90 degrees
- Repeat for 15-20 repetitions
- **TIP:** Don't let your knees go past your toes when in squatting position

MOUNTAIN CLIMBERS

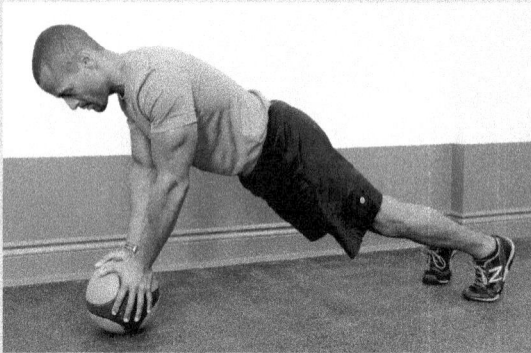

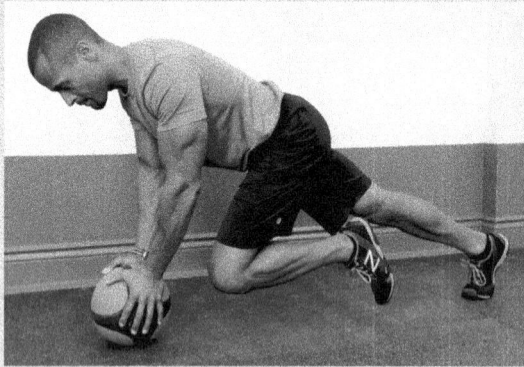

- Hands on floor or med ball and feet on the ground
- Move one knee towards the ball while keeping hips still and abs tight.
- Complete 20-30 repetitions (both knees = 1 rep)
- **TIP:** Don't let hips drop during the exercise

SQUAT WITH CHOP

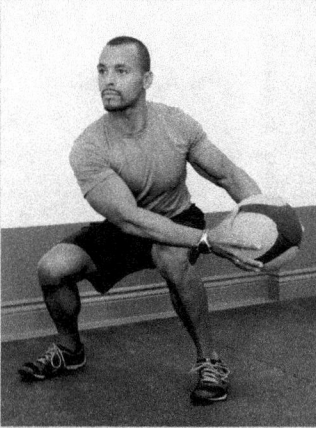

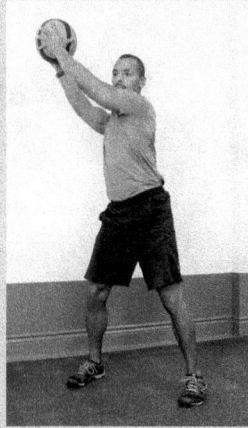

- Hold med ball or weight to one side while in squat position
- Come out of squat while quickly moving med ball upward diagonally
- Keep abdominal wall tight and arms straight
- Complete 15 each direction
- **TIP:** Keep your back straight and posture in correct form throughout exercise

TRIPOD

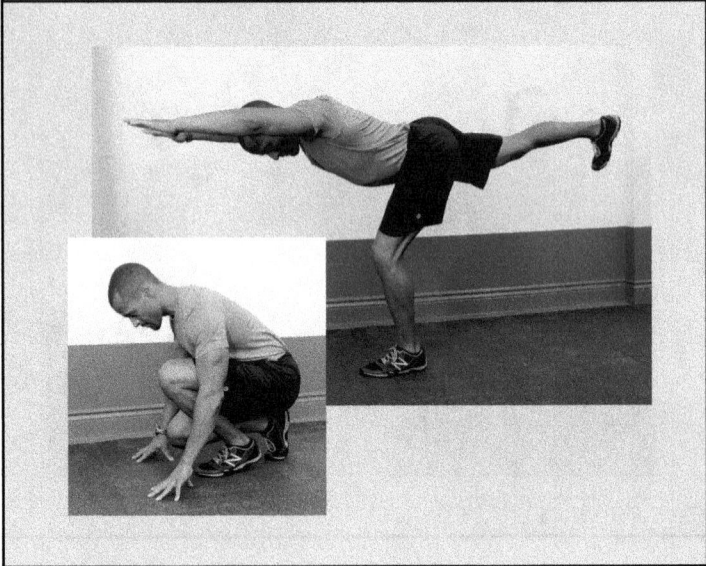

- Start in crouched position.

- Stand upright, pushing off one foot and extending the other backwards.

- Extend entire body parallel to the floor while balancing on the one leg.

- Repeat 10 repetitions, then move to opposite side

- **TIP:** Keep your head and neck in a neutral position

STARTER PROGRAM

LEVEL THREE *(Intermediate/Advanced)*

REQUIREMENTS:

- Complete 12 minutes of continuous running
- Distance score of 1.4 miles (2.25 km) or greater
- Greater than 15 Push Ups from the feet (women)
- Greater than 30 Push Ups from the feet (men)
- Greater than 2 minutes on the Abdominal Plank
- Greater than 2 minutes on the Wall Sit

PROGRAM DETAILS:

- Program Length: 6 weeks
- Duration: 30-40 minutes per workout, minimal rest between exercises.
- Frequency: 3 days per week plus 2 cardio days per week of 45-60 minutes

TOOLS REQUIRED:

- Dumbbells (12 – 45 lbs depending on ability)
  - *NOTE: Weight selection should be based on going to failure by the end of the required rep range and keeping form intact.*
- Fit ball
- Towel

WARM-UP

10 minutes skipping, jogging, cycling OR 10 minutes dynamic warm-up. For more information about sport-specific dynamic warm-ups and active stretching visit www.*IAmBishop.com/ThinkFactor*

COMPLETE 3 SETS

OF THIS 5 EXERCISE SEQUENCE

SQUAT THRUSTERS

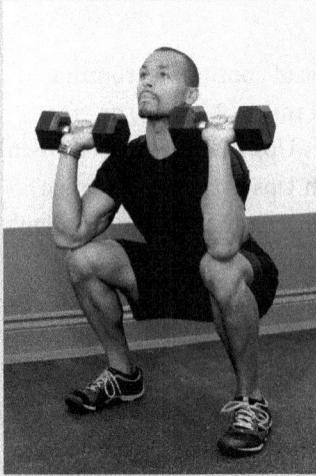

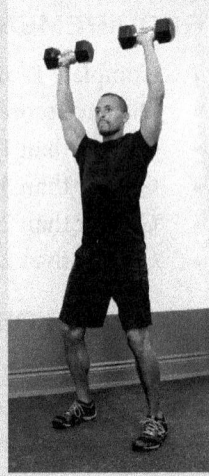

- Hold dumbbells with palms facing forward and elbows close together
- Sink down into squat with your weight on your heels
- Explosively power up out of squat while pressing above the head
- Complete 15 repetitions
- **TIP:** Generate speed and power from your legs to press the weights up. This ensures full body mechanics and lessens the work on the shoulders

RENEGADE ROW

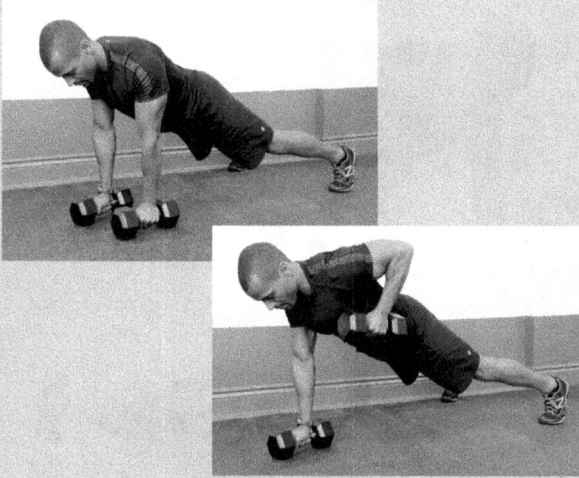

- Position dumbbells on ground slightly wider than shoulder width
- Position feet farther than shoulder width apart and hands on dumbbells
- While keeping core tight, explosively pull dumbbell up to arm pit
- Return to ground in a controlled manner then continue on other side
- Alternate sides until you complete 12-20 repetitions total
- **TIP:** Positioning feet farther apart will provide more stability through hips

PUSHUP WITH SINGLE ARM SLIDE OUT

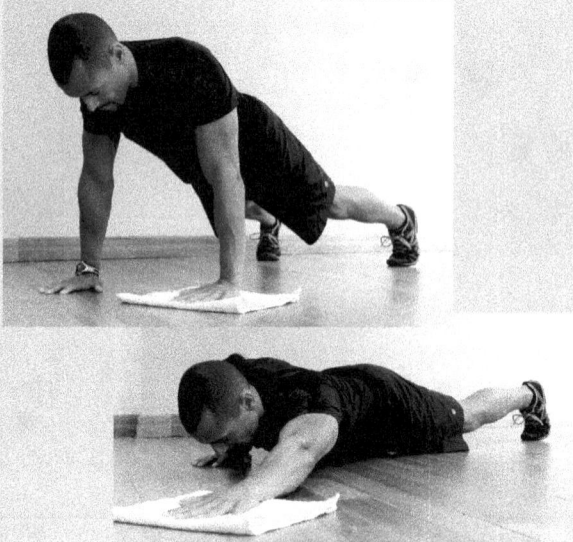

- In push up position, place one hand on towel
- Lower into push up while sliding one hand directly in front of you
- Exhale, come out of push up while pulling arm back into start position
- Complete 8-12 repetitions per side
- **TIP:** Keep core tight and hips straight. If hips are dropping decrease the reaching distance

LUNGE EXCHANGES

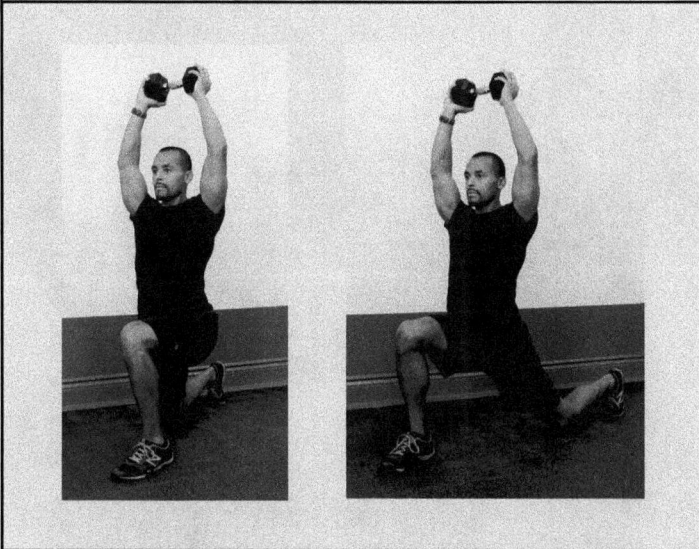

- Hold one dumbbell above head with straight arms
- Sink down into lunge position, keep back straight and core tight
- Explosively power up out of lunge and exchange leg positions
- Repeat the exchanges for 20-40 repetitions total based on ability
- **TIP:** Always absorb your landing through the front mid-foot

BODY SAW WITH TUCK

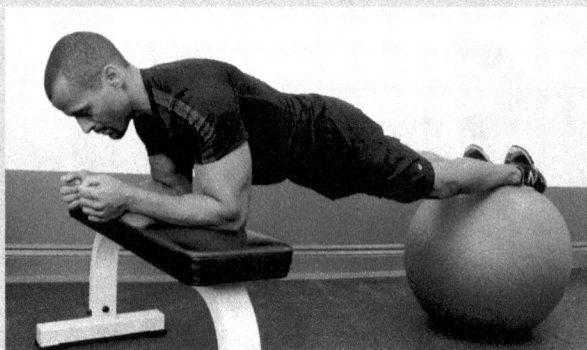

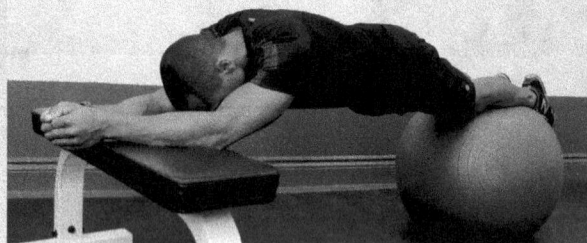

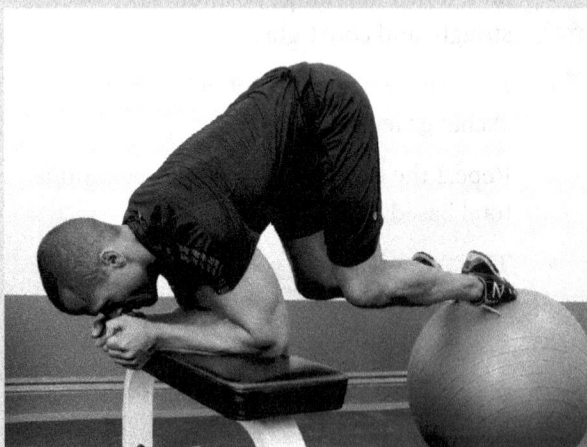

- Position forearms on bench and shins on fit ball
- Slowly hinge back from shoulders letting ball roll underneath your shins
- Exhale, returning back to original position and then tuck knees toward chest, contracting abdominals and raising hips upward
- Repeat this series for 10-20 repetitions based on form
- TIP: Do not let hips drop below parallel

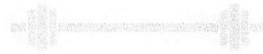

REMEMBER TO VISIT

www.IAmBishop.com/ThinkFactor

For unique and challenging ideas on how you can continue to progress to the next level, including more advanced workout routines, visit *IAmBishop.com/ThinkFactor.* Also, when you register on-line you receive access to one month of on-line coaching from me personally.

Chapter Seven

THE PLATEAU PHASE

There comes a point in everyone's life where their progress seems to flat line. This phase is called the Plateau, and it can be either short or prolonged. The reasons are different for everyone, but the fact remains—the Plateau is inevitable.

There are two ways to approach this phase. The wrong way is to accept it, stop growing and be defeated by it. The right way is to be aware of it, plan for it, minimize its duration, then blast right through it. The following stories illustrate this natural phase and how your approach and perspective can make a difference on how you get through it.

JUDY'S STORY

Judy had lost around 25 pounds when she hit her Plateau phase. She was much stronger, both physically and mentally than when she had started. It had been an amazing journey. However I could tell that something had shifted because the progress brought on by the change in stimulus seemed to have come to a dead halt. Not only was Judy no longer losing weight, but she had become hyper-focused on the fact that the number was not moving downward every time she got on the scale. She was pleased that it was not going up of course, but was having trouble accepting the fact that her weight loss was at a standstill. She had gotten used to losing weight fairly quickly.

It was the beginning of a new quarter, which meant it was time again to put Judy through a fitness evaluation. Every three months, we undergo a complete functional fitness evaluation that gives us a new benchmark on all areas of fitness—from body composition, to strength, to cardiovascular endurance and flexibility.

I remembered how much Judy had dreaded our very first fitness evaluation. Conversely she could hardly wait for the second evaluation because she knew just how far she had come and wanted to see the results on paper. We had completed a body composition test at around four and half months just to provide some motivation and prove she was in fact still on track compared to her third month benchmarks.

It was now Month 6. Although we had struggled during Month 1 while working on changing her mindset about the amount of effort required to get results. We had witnessed amazing results from Month 2 to about Month 5. Now she was at a point where the momentum had slowed down. I could tell that this was affecting Judy's performance and that she was becoming frustrated.

Judy had become extremely focused on losing weight, and despite seeing results in the areas of strength and endurance, we confirmed she was at a standstill in terms of losing additional body weight. It was time to shake things up a little, change the stimulus and try to redirect Judy's focus towards something tangible, experiential, and performance driven.

She was ready now for a new stimulus that would, in turn, move her off her current plateau. We decided on an event-based goal that required focused conditioning and preparation.

One spring day, after discussing her goals, we headed outside for a session. While we were warming up, I reminded Judy about the time when she had attempted to jog in her neighborhood. Also, that she had told me how she had been envious of those "skinny" people who could effortlessly take to the streets running when spring arrived.

After completing some warm up drills in the park, we were now going for a jog. At this point Judy was no longer a complete novice to jogging. She had done so for almost 20 minutes on the treadmill without stopping. The difference was that she had never really jogged outside.

As we began I noticed a change right away; she wasn't gasping for air or unable to talk while jogging. However, she was definitely disturbed. Her mind was telling her she couldn't do it. The change in her demeanor, mood and confidence was profound. After about four blocks Judy stopped in frustration, her eyes welling up with tears.

"I can't frickin' do this," she said. "I need to stop. I'm sorry, I'm sorry".

I asked why she thought she couldn't do it. Then I reminded her that she had jogged for almost 20 minutes in the gym and that she could breathe and talk while jogging. I told her it was her mind telling her she couldn't do it.

I suggested that she keep moving with a bounce in her step. It didn't matter how fast, but she had to keep on jogging very lightly.

After a pause, she started to jog again and every time I sensed she was going to stop, I said "keep bouncing, even if it is at a pace slower than walking. Get used to that feeling". I wanted her to get used to the movement, to being on the pavement, and to being outdoors. Then we could work on actually enjoying an activity that she once only dreamed about doing.

That day was very good for Judy. We must have run about two kilometres in all and I could see her expression of pride when we stretched out at the end of her session. She was glad she had not given up. To me, it was a small but powerful mental step that was just what she needed to push past her plateau.

TOM'S STORY

It was about one month before the half-marathon. Tom was progressing well with his run-conditioning program as we continued to work towards the event. By spending time strengthening his joints and increasing his flexibility, we were able to continue to increase his weekly distance without injury. He was motivated and pleased that he was able to work harder without pain.

To keep his muscles and tendons from tightening up, Tom had now acquired the habit of implementing regular stretching, massage therapy, and other myofacial release techniques (a form of soft tissue therapy). He was awed by the result—more movement; less pain.

Tom didn't achieve his personal best time when he ran the half-marathon. However, he was surprised and pleased by just how good he felt during the race, and by the fact that he was virtually pain-free after completing it. The run helped Tom realize just how important this more-sensible approach to exercise had been for him.

We were having our first session after he had completed the half-marathon. It was about mid-week. There was a sparkle in his eye, like that of a child who is up to something. He wanted my approval to push things a little harder and move a little quicker than the plan we had set out for him. He told me that he loved how he felt after completing the half-marathon and knew if he trained harder he would be able to achieve his personal best on the next race.

I was happy for Tom and glad to see him so excited about his progress. I also was aware of how he approaches life—all or nothing. Our next step in his program plan was a 60 kilometre mountain bike race that would take place in two months. This was another step towards his main goal, the three day competition, which would take place in about six months.

I continued to reiterate to Tom that in order to accomplish his main goal, it was important to take it step by step, achieving the mini goals we had set out at the beginning. In addition to maintaining his running, strength training and flexibility focus, we also introduced mountain biking to his program. For this, he was required to do a hill routine on his mountain bike once a week on his own. We would also meet each weekend to incorporate a longer, more technical, endurance ride.

Tom was eager. We planned to combine running with mountain biking on the same day. One morning he ran 21 kilometres on his own prior to starting a very technical mountain biking route. He got through about 20 kilometres before it came to an unfortunate end. I remember when I got the call.

"Brent, you're not going to believe this, I am out in the middle of nowhere lying in a ditch after hitting a stump, losing control and flying over top of my handle bars!"

He said this in an almost humorous way, but with a slightly painful laugh in his voice. Tom was strong, but I could tell he was in a lot of pain. After calling the paramedics, I drove to a location about one hour outside of the city to find him. He had broken his collarbone and suffered a Grade 3 tear of the **medial collateral ligament** (MCL) of his right knee. The MCL is one of the four major ligaments that help stabilize the knee.

We could never really say whether Tom was fatigued from pushing ahead too fast that morning or whether it was an accidental mishap. The reality however, was that he would now have to take several steps back in order to heal properly.

When unfortunate incidents like this happen, some people let the frustration get the best of them and give up. That's the wrong thing to do. We need to learn from the accident and focus on what we can do to recover and come back even stronger. That's the right thing.

This was a difficult plateau for Tom because it was not a natural fitness plateau but one forced upon him by this accident. Tom believed he was going to stagnate because of his inability to continue at this time. This was all the more frustrating because he had previously seen such significant results.

Tom's perspective had definitely been challenged. He became extremely frustrated. Although he began the required physiotherapy, his mind was not involved. He had given in to circumstances and succumbed to this plateau. It seemed like he had gone from all to nothing.

KIM'S STORY

As I reviewed Kim's training log and exercise history, it became apparent that her consistency over the past couple of months was questionable. An increasing number of last-minute cancellations; sometimes not showing up without notice, and longer delays on responding to my communications were all signs of someone who was slipping.

Either Kim had something going on in her personal life that was negatively affecting her lifestyle, or she had lost interest in exercise as a priority and integral component in her life.

I recall on several occasions trying to rebook her sessions and follow up with her, only to hear "Everything is great, I'm just so busy right now" or "I'm going to be focused and back on track next week". I knew she was regressing from the amazing results she had achieved.

Finally, I was able to schedule a session to sit down with Kim and discuss what was happening and why there was such inconsistency.

"Brent, I am at a low right now, a real low," she said. "I am finding it so challenging. I tried to get into volleyball again a while back and couldn't get into the league because it was full".

"I really felt like I was at a high—losing weight, feeling so energetic—but now I feel like I just don't have the drive to get through the workouts or even the day," she continued.

"This is exactly how I felt before we began, but after a couple of months of coming to see you regularly and doing your classes, I felt so good, like it was a part of my life. Now, mentally, I am really in a slump".

Now was the time to carefully re-examine how Kim's program related to her lifestyle, and to reflect on the past few months.

With the demands of her personal and professional life, Kim was going through a stage where not everything was clear. After being nominated for a Juno and receiving such great recognition, she felt that the spark from that high point was beginning to dwindle.

She had been through a great deal, both personally and professionally. She had lots of drive and passion for what she was doing, but she was having difficulty maintaining it. She had also shared with me the downside of not being represented by a professional manager. Often, having friends try to assist in this area was counterproductive to what she was trying to achieve.

"In many ways being a recognized artist in Canada is just not as effective as being recognized in the States," Kim explained to me in frustration.

The reason for Kim's fitness regression and current plateau was becoming increasingly clear—she lacked a life plan that would complement the vision she had for herself. She was well aware that making health and fitness brought her strength, confidence, and the resilience to deal with life's situations. However she had lost sight of that and allowed her mindset to shift. Having a clear sense of self and a vision for what you want out of life can provide enhanced focus and a positive energy that turns into results. At this point, my goal with Kim was to help her bring clear direction back into her life by helping her create a plan that would shift her current perspective. She needed to create a personal mission statement. A personal mission statement can be a powerful guide. It involves determining what you stand for (your core values), who you are as a person, and what you want to represent.

In addition, it was also apparent that for Kim to witness further results and get off the Plateau, she needed to change her perspective on nutrition. Not only did she need to learn more about what foods to avoid but also what foods would be highly beneficial for weight loss, performance, and energy. I suspected Kim also needed to be more truthful about her current diet. I wasn't confident that it was as clean as she said.

Once fitness improvements have taken effect, quite often nutrition becomes an increasingly important factor in significantly changing body composition. At the beginning of a lifestyle shift that incorporates regular exercise, while simultaneously carrying increased responsibilities like a new family, many people find it very difficult to make drastic changes in nutritional intake at the same time.

Kim's program initially focused on keeping her exercise purposeful and took a more subtle approach to her diet. Because the introduction of regularly scheduled exercise was challenging time-wise, it was all Kim could successfully handle.

Now that fitness had laid the foundation and jumpstarted her metabolism, Kim was ready for the next component—a nutrition overhaul. Armed with a personal mission statement, a new perspective, and a clearer life plan, the goal was to push her through the Plateau by keeping her motivated and accountable.

THE COMMON THREAD

Although the situations and experiences of Judy, Tom and Kim differ, they all eventually reached a Plateau. This is a common situation with those seeking my expertise in regards to toning, performance, and weight loss goals. One of the most common questions about the Plateau is:

"I am working out consistently, at least four days a week, but my weight has stopped going down—what's going on"?

First of all, let me assure you that this is a situation many people face when they try to lose weight. They find an activity they enjoy, begin implementing it regularly, see some initial results and then, for some reason, those results stop coming.

WHY DO WE REACH A PLATEAU?

Everyone experiences it differently, for different reasons and different durations. Following are three common reasons why it happens:

1. THE PSEUDO PLATEAU—WHAT DOES THE SCALE SAY?

I often come across what I call, the Pseudo Plateau. This is a common situation that can really wreak havoc with your motivation to keep to your plan. The weight scale may give the illusion that you are at a plateau; even though you are still attaining results. This is because the scale is generally not the best measurement of weight loss. All it tells you is your total body weight. A much more effective benchmark can be obtained by having your fitness professional test your body composition.

A body composition test will not only tell you your body fat percentage, but also how much of your weight is attributed to "fat weight" and how much is attributed to "lean weight" (muscle tissue, bone density, organs etc…).

Monitoring your body's progressive compositional change is a far more valuable benchmark. These statistics, along with basic girth measurements—such as arm girth, waist girth and thigh girth—give you a more accurate understanding of how your body is responding to your exercise and nutrition program.

Someone who is fairly new to exercise and strength training will always see an initial climb in lean weight, which tends to offset the drop in fat weight. Because of that, the overall change in total body weight (what the scale shows) can be very misleading. For example, someone could lose about 10 pounds in fat weight while gaining about eight pounds in lean weight. This is tremendous progress, but the scale will only show a two pound weight loss—discouraging for many.

So, what should you do to avoid the Pseudo Plateau from killing your motivation? Have your body composition tested by a fitness professional at the start of your program and at least every third month as you go along. In addition, don't discount the other amazing benefits that come along with regularly physical activity. Refrain from weighing yourself daily, understanding that you are achieving significant compositional changes and numerous health benefits in addition to weight loss.

2. PHYSICAL ADAPTATION

Reaching a physical plateau (or fully-adapted stage) during your exercise program can lead to a downturn in your exercise adherence and motivation to keep moving forward. This is usually the case for people who do not continue to challenge themselves in their exercise routines. Using physical challenge to bring transformational results in your life is powerful for weight loss or any other lifestyle goal.

What was difficult during the beginning stages of your exercise program becomes less difficult as your body adapts, and ultimately easy for you. The human body is remarkable in adapting to whatever stimulus it consistently receives. If that stimulus doesn't change over time, your body will reach complete physical adaptation. Continuing the same program may provide maintenance, but not change.

How do you ensure you are not coasting on a plateau? Two very effective tools that I use are:

❑ A JOURNAL/EXERCISE LOG

Using a Journal/Exercise Log daily to track your nutrition, how you feel, and your exercise progression can be a very effective way of ensuring that any plateau you hit is short-lived. Of course, the key to making this tool effective is by carefully reflecting on your journal entries, so that you can recognize patterns and the leveling off of results.

❑ A HEART RATE MONITOR

The use of a Heart Rate Monitor is one of the single most effective tools to maximize results and beat the plateau. Not only can you use it to track your progress and continue to push yourself, but most models also provide you with excellent feedback about calories burned, average heart rate, and maximum heart rate during each workout.

Use this feedback to provide yourself with some tangible goals to attain on your next workout. For example, burn 20 more calories than the previous workout or increase your average heart rate by five beats per minute.

For more information about Heart Rate Guided Training and choosing the right heart rate monitor for you and your goals, visit *www. IAmBishop.com/ThinkFactor* and register today.

3. MENTAL ADAPTATION

Like anything else, when an activity becomes predictable, it also becomes monotonous. Both the body and the mind fully adapt to repeated activity. Kim's story shows that this condition can be made worse by the lack of a fitness plan as well as an overall life plan. Lack of vision or direction can leave you with feelings of uncertainty, failure, and incapability. Personal life goals should be reviewed regularly and your exercise program should be completely overhauled at least every three months. In fact for best results, it is highly advantageous to have a different workout focus for each of your weekly training days. For example, Day 1 and Day 2 may have a running focus (one day hills and then other day distance) while Day 3 has a strength focus and Day 4 a core training focus.

You should also have weekly goals to keep moving yourself forward. This may entail increasing the amount of hill repeats, slightly increasing your distance, or trying to attain just two more repetitions on your strength days.

The common thread within the Plateau phase is the presence of little or no variability. This leads to a standstill or leveling off of results. For many people, a physical flat lining in results is usually followed by a mental plateau that can cause frustration and often halt your effort and commitment towards your fitness goal.

By sharing the stories in this chapter I hope to inspire you by explaining this inevitable phase, and to provide you with the tools to recognize it and help you be proactive in minimizing its duration.

Fit Tip

GENERAL NUTRITION TIPS

KEYS TO LOOKING LEAN AND FEELING GREAT

DON'T DRINK YOUR CALORIES

Stay away from sodas, moderate alcohol intake to less than 2-3 oz. per week, and minimize fruit juices. Eat fruit and other healthy snacks.

Sliced almonds, air-popped popcorn and a variety of fresh fruits and vegetables are great alternatives to processed snacks—get rid of baked goods, candies, and chocolates from your kitchen. These items are not only calorie dense, but contain far less nutritional value.

TRY YOGURT AS AN ALTERNATIVE

Great for a snack and a great alternative to higher fat cream based options. Skip the mayonnaise based dips and spreads. You can also use yogurt, instead of cream, to thicken sauces and soups. Every bit counts when it comes to cutting calories, and this is a great place to start if you are a dipper or spreader!

VEG OUT

Use vegetable purées as thickeners instead of meat or cream stocks for soups or cooking. This can give you the rich feeling without the fat and way less calories.

Battle the bloating

Reduce sodium intake by placing your salt shaker out of reach and try gluten free products to prevent bloating.

Hydrate Your Body

Virtually every process in your body is reliant on water and your muscles are 70% water. Imagine the detrimental effect on performance if you are constantly dehydrated. Science has proven that you will positively effect weight loss and maximize performance when you are consistently hydrated.

Daily Fit Tips For Healthy Weight Loss

❑ *Eat five times each day to maximize your metabolism*

❑ *To maximize weight loss, limit your carbohydrate intake to 20-30 grams at breakfast and lunch. Dinner should consist of protein and vegetables.*

❑ *Preplan your snacks for energy (ie; 12-15 almonds and a cup of yogurt)*

❑ *Limit alcohol consumption to 2 ounces or less per week*

❑ *Drink a minimum of 8 glasses of water each day*

Remember to Visit

www.IAmBishop.com/ThinkFactor

You'll receive access to useful worksheets, training guides, additional fitness programs and exclusive access to Brent Bishop for one month of free on-line coaching!

EATING FOR PERFORMANCE DAILY NUTRITION LOG

EXAMPLE BALANCED PLAN

MEAL 1 7:30 am	• scrambled egg with green pepper, wheat toast • coffee & 8oz orange juice • 1 glass of water
SNACK 10:00 am	• low fat fruit yogurt • apple • 10-15 almonds • 2 glasses of water
MEAL 2 12:30 pm	• whole wheat pasta salad with tuna, celery, peppers and carrots • 1 glass of water
SNACK 4:00 pm	• 1 cup yogurt with berries • 1 glass of milk • 2 glasses of water
MEAL 3 6:30 pm	• grilled salmon • asparagus • 1 glass of water
SNACK 8:30 pm	• 1 glass of water or herbal tea

EATING FOR PERFORMANCE
DAILY NUTRITION LOG

MY DAY

MEAL 1

_____
TIME

_____
_____
_____
_____

SNACK

_____
TIME

_____
_____
_____
_____

MEAL 2

_____
TIME

_____
_____
_____
_____

SNACK

_____
TIME

_____
_____
_____
_____

MEAL 3

_____
TIME

_____
_____
_____
_____

SNACK

_____
TIME

_____
_____
_____

Chapter Eight

THE BREAKTHROUGH PHASE

By demanding more of yourself, and then rising to that challenge, you can move yourself closer to your goals. This will soon become your new reality, leaving your former reality behind you.

Have you ever heard a speech that was so powerful, so unexpected, that it not only moved you immensely, but also changed your entire perspective in a matter of minutes?

Imagine being so exhausted from lack of sleep, working overtime and experiencing so much defeat from the general stresses of life that you can't see yourself doing anything but sleeping when you have a day off. Now imagine that just as you're about to turn in for the night, you get an unexpected call from an old time college friend who is in town for just one day and wants to get together with you. The result is an instantaneous shift in your mindset. In an instant you are alert, excited and ready to change your plans completely.

This is the power of the mind, a power that can be harnessed in mere seconds. When an event causes you to shift your perspective, alter your current frame of mind, and focus inspired energy to take action, you are experiencing "the Breakthrough". This state of mind most commonly occurs by an unplanned or unexpected event. However, it is possible to consciously create such a breakthrough, sustain it, and see it through to the attainment of your goals.

Most athletes are highly focused. This ability to direct their mindset is what drives them to success. This ability is what you need to demand more of yourself and maximize your potential in every area of your life. You must know yourself inside and out. Awareness of what inspires you and how to maximize that inspiration through purposeful challenge, as well as how to proactively manage those things that may go wrong and cause you to falter.

Judy, Tom and Kim each had a different perspective, and they all managed, in separate ways, to reach the Breakthrough phase.

JUDY'S STORY

Judy was somewhat frustrated because she was still at a plateau in her weight loss journey. Sharing with her some of the experiences I'd had with other clients put her mind more at ease and started her to hope again. The previous week I had challenged her mind by getting her to run outdoors. I say "challenged her mind" because her fitness level was not the problem. She was actually quite well conditioned at this point in her program. She was tough enough to handle an hour-long intense boxing session without stopping.

The problem was that she had developed a mental block that defeated her the previous week. When she felt her feet on the pavement, the mental scenario she believed for years returned— that only "skinny" people could run outside. She assumed that she was going to be embarrassed because she wouldn't be able to do it.

I saw this as an opportunity to once again challenge what was most important, what spurred her to action, success, and continued weight loss. She needed to shift her mindset about what was possible and to convince herself that she was a runner, and that she was actually good at it. With her trust and cooperation we could get her off her current plateau. Then she could reach beyond what she initially thought that she was capable of. I was on board and committed. I just needed to convince her to be the same.

Quite often, others see potential in you that you are unable to see in yourself. Sometimes all you need is a little push.

After telling Judy my plan, we headed outside to continue where we had left off the previous week. It was not enjoyable, and to make matters worse, it was raining.

Judy stopped herself again and again, giving in to self-defeat. We tried three more times over the next few sessions, and although each was slightly better than the previous one, there was still not a lot of progress. I felt Judy was beginning to resent me and my plan.

"Brent, I am honestly not that into running," she said to me as we walked back into the studio after a morning run/walk routine. "I just feel really heavy, unfit and disappointed in myself. I thought I wanted to be able to run, but it's not that important to me now that I know what it feels like. I would be happy to continuing doing more boxing for my cardio—I love that".

I didn't want to ignore what she wanted, but stopping just before she was about to break through would only lend credence to her belief that she was not a runner—that she was out of shape and unfit. We would have to continue to try to break through this mindset or find a new way to get her beyond the plateau.

I had reviewed her workout journals and reflected on the notes from the consultation we'd had six months before. There was no doubt that one of her recurring goals was to "be able to take advantage of a beautiful day by going out for a run".

The very next day, I sat her down prior to our workout and reviewed these details with her. I read the exact words she said about two weeks into her program "I wish I could run, but running is for skinny people". I could tell this struck a chord as she tried to mask the onset of tears. Reflection is powerful. Judy admitted that in fact this was still her desire but she didn't feel capable of achieving it. However, she said she was open to discussing how we could get her there.

As she continued to incorporate boxing and the other elements that Judy enjoyed into her weekly routine, we also created a tighter plan for her running that culminated with a five-kilometre race six weeks from now. The idea of competing in a race was nerve racking for her. It was a definite mental and physical challenge, but she moved forward with the plan.

As the weeks passed, it became evident that her mindset towards running, and her level of confidence were changing. Judy was now able to run continuously for about 20 minutes— outside. The turnaround had begun.

Two weeks prior to the race we did a trial run to familiarize Judy with the route. It went well. She had to stop a few times where there was a slight incline in the route, but overall she accomplished what she came out to do. Although she was a little upset with herself for stopping part way through, she was content that she had familiarized herself with the course.

Race day: at 6:30 am I checked my voicemail. There was a message from Judy.

"I don't feel so well today," she said. "I really hate to do this but I don't think I can meet you for the race. Maybe, there will be another one later in the summer that I can do…"

"This is nothing but an excuse," I thought to myself. Fear of taking on a challenge was either going to haunt her for the rest of her life or help her accomplish one of the most monumental fitness goals she had created for herself—to become a runner.

There was more wrapped up in this event than weight loss. This was to be her moment to shine; to prove to herself that she was capable of much more than she had initially thought. I was not going to let her throw this opportunity away.

The race was set to start at 8:00 am. After eating a quick breakfast, I rushed out of the house, drove directly to her place and, knocked on her door.

"Got your message and just wanted to see how you were feeling," I said to her. She could tell I didn't believe her message. She admitted that, once again, fear was getting the best of her.

Agreeing to go with me, Judy made her way step-by-step, breath-by-breath—never stopping even once—straight through to the end of her very first running race. A look of complete exhilaration came across her face as she pushed harder for those last few meters, hearing the crowd. As her feet crossed that finish line, I will never forget the tears of joy, sense of accomplishment and pride in Judy's eyes as she raised her hands in the sky trying to regain her breath.

That day Judy became a runner. She committed to her goal, conquered her fears and placed herself into the same category as those "skinny people" who were able to "enjoy a beautiful day by going out for a run". This was the Breakthrough for Judy and this was the moment that changed her life, her outlook and her awareness that she could accomplish anything she put her mind to.

TOM'S STORY

After some physiotherapy we were able to continue working on Tom's rehab and strength development. The results were now more noticeable. The challenge was to keep Tom focused mentally on what was required—what he could do at the present time and where he was heading. The knee was healing remarkably well. We were able to push hard on the spin bike and continue to focus on strengthening and stabilizing his knee. Although Tom's fitness was set back by his injury, he had stayed focused on the positives.

As a lead up to his big race in Colorado, the original plan was for Tom to enter a 60 kilometre bike race that would take place in three weeks. Tom's recovery was coming along well but I wasn't sure if it would be wise for him take part in this highly technical race. Knowing how competitive Tom was, the last thing I wanted was to have him re-injure himself.

So instead of entering the bike race, we decided to work towards full recovery of his knee and shoulder, by focusing his energy on the kayak race in two and half months. He could then do a 60-kilometre bike route when he had fully recovered.

Progress was being made. We were able to get onto the water weekly and introduce more paddling into his routine. This variation in routine not only allowed his body to recover, but also kept him mentally focused and motivated. We had reintroduced running, maintained his bike training, and continued to pick up distance on his paddling.

Although Tom experienced some discomfort from time to time, he was able to push forward, increasing his focus on muscular balance and flexibility, while conditioning himself for his upcoming events.

Tom was beginning to feel stronger and becoming increasingly excited about his main goal, the Colorado competition in four months. The morning of his kayak race was gloomy but warm. When the participants were setting up, the water was so still that it resembled glass. Tom's energy was great, his body conditioned and his mind focused. He was poised and alert in his start position at the countdown.

Immediately after the horn blew, the glass-like surface of the water shattered as nearly 50 paddles cut through its surface simultaneously. It was amazing to watch. Tom took off without hesitation; the power behind his paddling seemed unmatchable. The true challenge for Tom would be his level of endurance— would he be able to maintain a pace that would keep him on top for over 15 kilometres?

That day Tom finished in the Top 10. He was pleased and was back on track. Meanwhile, the big day was getting closer. Tom may have been set back by his injury, but at this point you would have never known.

The week of the Colorado event finally arrived and we anxiously boarded the plane about 20 hours before we had to be at the starting line. On the flight to Denver, Tom told me how happy he was with his progress after the accident; how he never thought he would get to this point so soon. I could tell he was very excited and was confident that he would do well. I was going to compete along with him, which in itself would be a challenge for me.

It was around 70 degrees that morning, the air was still and the sun was just rising. All the participants were either lined up or warming up as we all anxiously awaited the start of the race. The start was strong. Tom and I began at a steady pace; keeping in mind that pacing would be crucial to success. He was feeling great, and my goal was to keep up with him and give him coaching tips along the way.

His performance in the run was amazing and we successfully made the transition onto the mountain bikes and began our ascent on the first hill. My legs felt like lead and I knew Tom was feeling the same. At this point the unobstructed mid-morning sun was beginning to have an effect on our body temperatures. Keeping well hydrated was going to be important to avoid cramping up. From gravel hill climbs to technical single-track trails, we managed to maintain our position in the biking portion despite being exhausted. At this point, I was also thankful I had put in my own training along with Tom. The terrain was not easy.

We were nearing our final leg of the day. It was the point where we got off the bikes and continued on foot. The grade of the mountain made it impossible to run this section regardless of whether we could have found the energy to run. Despite having a small error in our compass navigation, we ended the day well before the cut off time and were happy with our achievement.

Day 2 began with the relief of downhill running as we made our way back to the base of the mountain. Although it took us nearly two hours to traverse down the windy trails, it was a pleasant break from the uphill experience the day before. At the bottom, came our first paddling challenge. We were required to portage our kayaks for what felt like almost a kilometre through uneven rocky terrain to meet the water's edge.

We paddled through the relatively calm waters at a consistent pace for over two hours before hitting our final transition point that required us to portage uphill for about 200 meters. Then we would be at a trailhead where our bikes had been transported.

Day 2 ended about one and a half hours later than Day 1, Tom's knee was now experiencing some swelling and we were both exhausted, ready to eat dinner, and get some well deserved sleep.

It was Day 3. We had iced Tom's knee regularly to manage swelling and it seemed to be in good condition. This final day would take us approximately seven hours to complete beginning with a three-hour mountain bike trek consisting of various inclines and technical trails. Then there was a very strenuous trail running segment with navigation requirements, and finally an exhausting paddle in the kayaks to our last checkpoint before the finish line. The kayaking was grueling as the pressure was on to maintain our position in the race. It was apparent to everyone that the end was approaching and that every ounce of effort would count at this point.

After reaching the shoreline and dragging our kayaks out of the water, we had to portage uphill to the final challenge—scaling a 20-foot wall. The kayaks at this point felt like they weighed 300 pounds and our arms were exhausted from powering through the water. Tom and I reached the wall almost simultaneously, out of breath and almost collapsing from fatigue. From here it was teamwork, we continued to help each other up the wall, one of us scaling while the other assisted with strategically placed platforms and ropes. The feat seemed impossible, but we knew it could be done because we saw others conquer the wall and scream with exhilaration at the top.

After slipping a few times and pausing from loss of strength, we managed to conquer this final obstacle with absolutely nothing left but a pure sense of achievement as, catching our breath, we gazed at the 360 degree view of the mountain range.

The feeling was unbelievable—from a weekend warrior who was in constant chronic pain, to a determined athlete with an action plan, to an injured and unmotivated ex-athlete, to a revitalized competitor who had overcome all these setbacks to finish a grueling adventure race that epitomized success for him.

Through the journey that brought him to this point, Tom came to the realization that nothing is impossible. With an effective plan and the will to demand more of yourself, you can unleash your inner athlete and continue to achieving your goals.

KIM'S STORY

"Inspire the world with my voice and be a positive role model for my children through my actions and positive energy".

Kim now had a personal mission statement that stated who she was, what she stood for, and what she wanted out of life. The goal now was to get her to actually live it out consistently. Just like anyone, Kim would slip, whether it was her nutrition, her exercise consistency, or just keeping her word. We are all human and we will all fall sometimes, but the important thing is to have people in our lives that hold us accountable for our actions, remind us who we are and what we are capable of achieving in life. Without this, we are left to our own devices and sometimes that can be detrimental.

If you have a personal mission statement—a vision for your life—it will always be that beacon to get you back on track to where you want to be. If you habitually refer to it, your chances of success are great. If you share it with others who are close to you, they too can remind you of it when you are at a low point.

This was my plan for Kim. When she would forget to follow through with what she said by missing a workout or forgetting to send her nutrition log to me, I would simply recite her personal mission statement to her.

Once she was going through a tough week. Everything seemed to be going wrong. Her schedule was unmanageable, her expectations too high, her children misbehaving, she was irate from receiving a parking ticket, and then late for her training session—furious, frantic and filled with negative energy.

"Inspire the world with my voice and be a positive role model for my children through my actions and positive energy," I said after patiently listening to her vent. Immediately, I got a smile, a sigh and an instant shift in energy as the words of her personal mission statement reentered her mind, changing her emotional state. We then laughed it off and had a great focused workout that brought her stress level back down. Each time something like that happened, she would realize why she was committed to exercise. It wasn't just the weight loss but, more importantly, the impact it had on her well-being, her career focus, her relationships, and her ability to be that positive role model for her children.

As Kim continued her program, the occasions when I would have to remind her of her personal mission statement became more infrequent. Finally she was able to bring herself into the present moment without my intervention, thereby preventing unfortunate events and circumstances from defining her.

A few months after initiating the process of living by a personal mission statement and creating goals based upon it, Kim began working towards her Bachelor of Arts Degree. The unpredictability of her singing career had always been something that plagued her and she had a true interest in psychology. She knew singing and writing was her passion and she had so much to say in her music to inspire people, but she always had a deep desire to earn her degree. At some point she had given up that goal, thinking she couldn't do both. In fact she could.

It is now two years into her educational journey and she is not only enjoying the process but also, with physical health being a major priority, is not afraid to boast that she is in the best shape of her life both physically and mentally. Kim fully embodies her personal mission statement and it continues to represent who she really is. Her classes are providing valuable knowledge, she is married with a beautiful family, and continues to receive opportunities to write music and perform regularly with well-known artists. With a focused and meaningful plan, her actions continue to bring success and a future that is no longer guided by circumstance, but created with purpose.

THE COMMON THREAD

Each of these success stories involves the arrival of the Breakthrough, a moment triggered by an event, a progressive overcoming of adversity or challenge, and a point at which a permanent internal change has occurred. This internal change is so profound that there truly is no turning back. The interesting thing about the progression from the Dreamer phase to the Breakthrough phase is that once the momentum is created and you seek to find inspiration in everything you do, the process becomes continuous, growth inevitable, and you truly become the author of your life story.

In each of these stories you will notice that there are moments of new experiences that allow for a constant variety of stimuli that shift perspectives and let the individuals begin to see themselves and their circumstances in a different light. One of the most important factors in achieving the Breakthrough is knowing that your experiences can lead to positive changes in your life.

We all have preconceived views of the world, our capabilities within it and what is possible for us to achieve. Have you ever travelled to a country that you knew very little about, other than what has been portrayed to you through the media, friends and society? If so, you have probably noticed that after spending some time in that country, many of the ideas you may have had about its people, customs, and ways of living were inaccurate. Upon returning home, you have a new understanding and a completely different perspective about that country and its people. This is a new framework from which you cannot go backwards. You can no longer speak, think, or talk from the frame of reference you had prior to visiting that country.

This is a simple concept, but if you think about it, this new experience has a profoundly permanent result—it has changed the way you think. This kind of change allows you to educate others and speak from your new frame of reference. Having such an experience alters your actions, even if the alteration is so small that it is unnoticeable unless consciously reflected upon.

Progress in health, fitness and positive lifestyle change is not much different from this example. In my opinion, creating a purposeful experience in your life is the number one way to learn—a way that is meaningful, insightful, and lasting. Each experience will provide a small breakthrough in some way, whether it is how you interact with someone, the energy you give off to others and your surroundings, or the actions you take when you first wake up in the morning. If your actions are properly planned and interest-driven, you have the capability to create your own profound physical and mental experiences through fitness and active living. They are what lead you to the Breakthrough—one of the most important transitions you will ever make.

Fit Tip

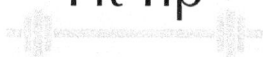

5 Ways to Trigger your Think Factor during Exercise

1. Get Inspired

Exercise for some is tough enough to start as it is. If find you are forcing yourself to do activities that you just don't have an interest in—you are going in the wrong direction.

You can't do anything successfully in life without being inspired to do it. If you are not inspired, you cannot be motivated. Making sure you first seek to be inspired in your fitness endeavors will ensure you get started with momentum.

It may be going outdoors, trying out a new class or watching an inspiring movie—just start with inspiration and your path will begin to become clearer.

2. Pre-Visualization

A high level athlete, whether they are a downhill skier, sprinter or cyclist will actually visualize the entire race in their mind before they practice or race the route. Not only will they visualize the route but also they will visualize themselves winning, crossing that finish line with feelings of euphoria. These feelings are so real that every sense in their body experiences it.

Why is this so important for success? The mind is the most powerful tool in the world. Your thoughts control every action you do, and your mindset and attitude can either set you up for success or failure. Which will you choose?

3. MUSICAL EMOTION

There is something about music, particularly that artist, that beat, that song which intrinsically changes your body's chemistry. It can take a feeling of low energy and propel it to the highest of heights.

Make a playlist that motivates and emotionally inspires you to "get it done". This will maximize your efforts during your workout.

4. VISUAL THINKING

Exercise is physiologically complex. We are placing our body, its muscles, its neurological system and its joints under stress in complex ways in order to achieve the results we desire. If you are not attentive to the movement of your body, you are not present. If you are not present, you are not maximizing your form and concentrating your efforts on the task at hand.

Do you ever catch yourself reading a book or article only to realize minutes after that your mind was drifting and you can barely recall the content you have just read about? Visual thinking during exercise can help concentrate your efforts on what you are doing and assist your muscular and neurological system to work in unison efficiently. It may be visualizing the muscle contract when you are working it, imagining your muscles lengthen as you stretch them, or muscles relaxing as you exhale with long breaths. Or it may be envisioning your sports idol getting that winning goal or pushing that final distance. The point is, we all have visual triggers that allow us to push further and perform better.

5. THE 2-REP-RULE OR 15-SECOND-RULE

If you've ever worked with a trainer, participated in a class where you were motivated, or been part of a sports team; you will be familiar with the phenomenon of being able to perform at a higher level than you do when you're alone. This is human nature.

Alone, we will generally give up quicker, come up with excuses sooner, and demand less of ourselves. When we are accountable to others, we perform better. This occurs even with a very non-competitive person. There is a way to enhance your solo effort. It involves setting targets before you start and sticking to them while you are exercising.

Generally speaking, you can always do 2 more reps, hold 15 seconds longer, or do slightly more than you initially think you can. Think about it—if your life depended on it would you hold an exercise for 15 more seconds to stay alive?

Placing a realistic target for yourself will guarantee progress with your exercise plan.

REMEMBER TO VISIT

www.IAmBishop.com/ThinkFactor

When you register on-line you receive access to one month of on-line coaching from me personally and access to my special fitness and lifestyle tools, including three complete individualized programs that will guide your progress. You can register anytime by visiting *www.IAmBishop.com/ThinkFactor*

Chapter Nine

SURPASS YOUR EXPECTATIONS

Because we are all different, our individual characteristics and circumstances exert differing influences on our personal lifestyles. This, in part, can account for why some of us achieve fitness results faster than others.

The three stories in this book illustrate three different situations. The common theme with Judy, Tom and Kim was that in the end they did not give up. Like anyone on a journey that involves change, each of them became discouraged at times.

As with Judy, Tom and Kim, you will likely stray from your plan occasionally. However being aware of this right from the start, and having the tools to manage your life, are two of the essential elements of perseverance.

In the beginning of this book, I explored the idea of abandoning mediocrity, leaving behind the acceptance of what society deems as "have to's" and "should be's". I wrote about the importance of having a dream and going for it, moving in the direction of your inspiration and being persistent so you can achieve what you desire.

Because you have the ability to change, it is of great importance to reflect on what you need to do in order to realize your dreams, as well as how essential it is that you take ownership of your actions.

Next, we examined who you truly are at present and who you want to be in the future. We discussed the importance of initiating an action plan to get to your destination and how to develop new habits that you can build upon. Habitual actions help form and develop character, and through character changes you become what your actions represent. This is true progress.

I discussed how The Performance Continuum Paradigm© relates to your life and your goals in a systematic way to ensure that you are aware of your actions. This enables you to move forward with purpose. It also provides you with a practical model of accountability with which you can track your progress.

Now that you are aware of the essential steps required to form your action plan, and a summary of what you can expect to encounter on your journey, it will be beneficial to take some time to review The Performance Continuum Paradigm© on the next page.

Spending time reviewing this paradigm and reflecting on how it applies to you, will increase the clarity of the vision that you have for your fitness and lifestyle goals. You may also want to revisit Chapter 3 to familiarize yourself again with the explanation of how this important model is interpreted.

The idea of continuously and purposefully extending your comfort zone, both to broaden who you are as a person and also to introduce challenge into your life, is an important theme throughout this book. Whether you are in the Dreamer, Doer, Plateau or Breakthrough phase, it is important to realize that this is an ongoing process.

THE PERFORMANCE CONTINUUM PARADIGM©

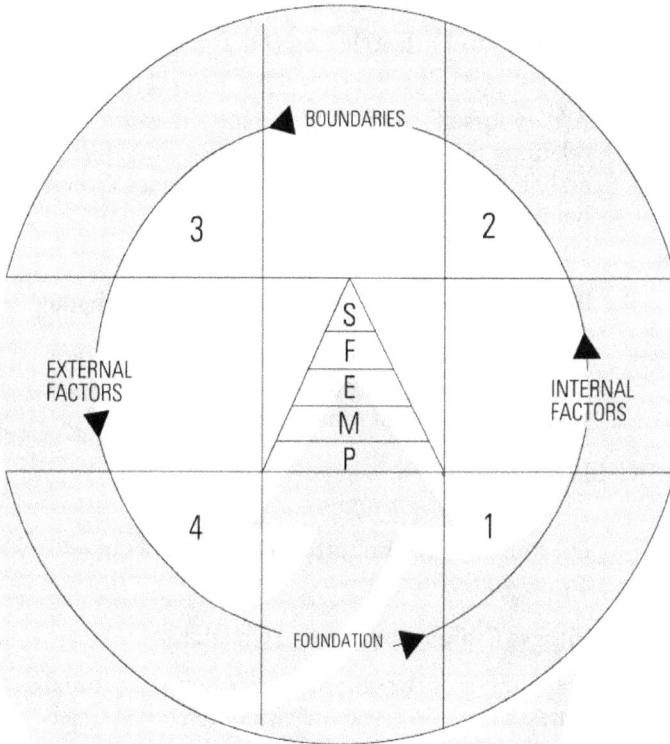

Now that you have taken the journey through the stories outlined in the previous chapters and have begun some of the fundamentals of creating momentum through fitness, it's an opportune time to tie it all together and tighten up your action plan. What follows is a step-by-step checklist to revisit your action plan and tailor it to reflect your new level of understanding.

1. REVISIT & REVIEW THE GROUND WORK

Take the time to review the exercises you have completed within the previous chapters of this book:

A. **Exercise and Lifestyle Log** (Fit Tip: Chapter 1)
   Register online to receive your free copy of this Log

   Ask yourself some important questions in relation to your review of your log. What activity(s) were you able to change so far? Which habits are holding you back and which moving you forward?

B. **Inspiration Identity Worksheet** (Fit Tip: Chapter 2)

   In your review of this worksheet, are you now consciously doing more activities that inspire you rather than ones that do not inspire you?

C. **Life Strategy Worksheet** (Fit Tip: Chapter 3)
   Register online to receive your free copy of this Log

   Do your Areas of Importance reflect more of what you are now prioritizing?

D. **Fitness Evaluation** (Fit Tip: Chapter 4)

   Depending on when you completed your initial fitness evaluation, you may want to retest yourself now and see if you score higher.

   If you began with Starter Program Level One, you may find that your evaluation score now shows that you have progressed to Starter Program Level Two. If this is the case, congratulations— you are progressing physically!

   If you haven't yet worked with the program for about a month, not to worry—stay consistent and you will begin to see progress.

   You should do a re-evaluation every three months at a minimum, however initially you may retest after one month to see how you are performing. If you have been consistent, you are likely to see some gains in performance.

E. **Starter Program** (Fit Tip: Chapter 6)

If you began with Starter Program Level One and found that when you performed the Fitness Evaluation again you have now attained a score that suggests you do Starter Program Level Two—now's the time to switch. If you find you have progressed beyond Starter Program Level Two, then you can begin Starter Program Level Three. If you find you have progressed beyond Starter Program Level Three, visit *www. IAmBishop.com/ThinkFactor* and request additional programs.

Remember: when you register on-line you will receive one month of on-line coaching from me personally, and access to my special fitness and lifestyle tools. This includes three completely individualized programs that will guide your progress to your next Breakthrough.

F. **General Nutrition Tips** (Fit Tip: Chapter 7)

Take another look at the Nutrition Tips suggested and familiarize yourself with them, as nutrition can play an integral role in your rate of success.

G. **5 Ways to Trigger Your Think Factor During Exercise** (Fit Tip: Chapter 8)

Review these useful tips to ensure that you are maximizing your efforts during your workouts.

2. CREATE YOUR PERSONAL MISSION STATEMENT

This statement should be succinct, clear and encapsulate who you are, what you value, and what you stand for in life. Think of this statement representing who you have become in the future but written in the present tense. For example, in Kim's story she had created a personal mission statement as follows: "Inspire the world with my voice and be a positive role model for my children through my actions and positive energy".

3. FEED YOUR LIFE COMPONENTS

In The Performance Continuum Paradigm©, the center triangle outlines the "Pyramid of Self". These five components (Physical, Emotional, Mental, Financial, and Spiritual) all play some role in your life. It is important to identify how you "feed" these areas of fitness (the source) to ensure that you are not neglecting one or more of these components.

Being physically active and nutritionally aware will act as a vehicle to success in all areas of your life. However, you must also remember to allot time to all areas as they are equally important. For example, regular visits with a good friend or partner may feed your emotional fitness; spending time each week to read and educate yourself in new areas is a good way to feed your mental fitness; having a sound investment plan like contributing regularly to a retirement fund can help feed your financial fitness.

Spiritual fitness, like the other areas, can be different for everyone. Perhaps for you it is scheduling regular walks through the forest or simply meditating daily, praying, or listening to enlightening music. The main point is, find what works for you personally, what inspires you deeply, and prioritize this into your personal action plan to ensure a balance in your life.

4. OUTCOME PLANNING (DETERMINE YOUR O.P.P.)

Outcome, Purpose Statement and Plan of Action: for goals to become attained, conceptualizing them as outcomes can be quite effective. A goal can be seen as a desire or a goal to be achieved. An outcome, on the other hand, is an actual result. Start with long-term outcomes (i.e., 1-5 years) then work backward to create short-term outcomes (i.e., quarterly, monthly, etc.) that lead up to the long term ones.

Additionally, to bring purpose to your long and short-term outcomes, create a purpose statement that coincides with the outcome. This will create the meaning and passion that will enable your momentum.

I have included some examples on the following pages to better illustrate this powerful process.

Here's an example

Main Outcome = Marathon, 2013

- Purpose:

  Decrease body fat by 10%, increase cardiovascular fitness, sense of accomplishment

- Purpose Statement:

  To optimize my health and wellness and be in the best shape of my life

- Plan of Action:

  Long Term:

  > July 14th, 2013—Marathon

  Short Term:

  > March 1st, 2013—½ Marathon
  > January 15th, 2013—10 km Race

- Time Management:

  - Use a Day Planner or Planning Software
    - (Quarterly, Monthly, Daily tracking/planning)
  - Weekly Exercise Routine (see next page)
  - Corresponding nutrition regimen with daily food log
  - Scheduled weekly review and reflection

EXAMPLE WEEKLY EXERCISE ROUTINE

5 DAY A WEEK RUNNER'S ROUTINE

Monday	Recovery Run 30 minutes
Tuesday	60 minutes Full Body Strength
Wednesday	Hill Repeats (6-10 times, 200 meters each)
Thursday	REST DAY
Friday	60 minutes Full Body Strength
Saturday	REST DAY
Sunday	Long Run—60+ minutes (build distance weekly)

To successfully achieve fitness results and a profound lifestyle change will take some people longer than others. Focusing on building your inner strength and enlisting a strong support system can have dramatic outcomes. Using physical fitness and positive lifestyle choices is your vehicle to true and powerful change that can successfully transform your perception of your own capabilities.

Step by step, you will become stronger, more confident, possess greater energy, enhance your focus, and exude these changes to those around you. Time and again in my work, I have seen dramatic physical changes of weight loss and athletic development. More importantly, I have seen changes of character, mindset, and personal perception, changes that are far greater than any physical change. In fact, it is due to these profound changes in character that weight loss and fitness results were realized and maintained.

When you are able to find that spark—that inner drive—that ignites who you are as a person (your inner athlete), you will ultimately create the momentum that will take you far beyond what you had initially planned for yourself.

The Breakthrough phase will be a milestone and you will realize that you have been propelled to a new perception of yourself, developed new capabilities, and achieved profound and meaningful results. This doesn't happen by magic, but by consciously determining what you want and systematically working to obtain it.

You will have reached your destination because you followed your inspiration, welcomed the challenge and did not take no for an answer. You will have arrived at a time in your life when you can no longer be trapped in the past, a time when it is impossible to revert back to the way you were, and a time when new breakthroughs are continually being created.

You will have found your Think Factor.

Fit Tip

REMEMBER TO TAKE ADVANTAGE OF MY ADDED BONUSES!

Visit
www.IAmBishop.com/ThinkFactor

When you register on-line you receive access to one month of on-line coaching from me personally and access to my special fitness and lifestyle tools, including three complete individualized programs that will guide your progress. You can register anytime by visiting *www.IAmBishop.com/ThinkFactor*

Glossary

ACTION PLAN (OR PLAN OF ACTION)

A weekly or daily summary of the action items that allows you to stay on track with your overall long-term plan.

HABIT

A behavior, or pattern of behaviors, that becomes a regular part of repeated routine.

HEART RATE MONITOR

A tool comprised of a chest strap and a watch receiver that provides feedback on your heart rate and workout intensity.

INNER ATHLETE

The drive within every person which, when revealed and unleashed, inevitably produces profound physical and mental improvements in that person's life.

LIFE STRATEGY

The notion of proactively planning and devising a series of actions to accomplish what you want in life.

MYOFACIAL RELEASE TECHNIQUE

A form of soft tissue therapy used to treat whole body dysfunction and its resulting pain and restriction of motion. This encompasses a variety of techniques used to (i) increase circulation, (ii) loosen adhesions and thickening of the sheath that covers muscle, (iii) increase your rate of healing, and (iv) reduce the occurrence of musculoskeletal injury.

OPTIMAL PERFORMANCE

An individual's highest possible level of performance in any area of life.

O.P.P.

Outcome, Purpose Statement, Plan of Action: the three key components to planning for effective goal attainment.

PERFORMANCE CONTINUUM PARADIGM

A practical model for healthy living that is rooted in the notion of using physical health as the vehicle to life success.

PERSONAL MISSION STATEMENT

A descriptive statement established with the purpose of guiding your actions. The Personal Mission Statement encompasses your core values, what you stand for in life, and what defines you.

PSEUDO PLATEAU

A stage within a weight loss program whereby the individual feels they have reached a plateau (no longer seeing their body weight decline on the scale), however; they are in fact still losing fat weight while their lean weight (muscle tissue, bone density) has been increasing. In this situation the scale is deceiving, as it does not differentiate between lean weight and fat weight.

REFLEXIVE LEARNING

Learning that occurs automatically. Behaviors must be learned and automatic learning to specific circumstances within an individual's upbringing can be so strongly ingrained due to repetition.

TRAINING MODALITY

Any specific mode of training, for example cycling for a bike race, or hill sprints for run training.

www.ingramcontent.com/pod-product-compliance
Lightning Source LLC
Chambersburg PA
CBHW070252290326
41930CB00041B/2463